The Savvy Diabetic

A Survival Guide

The Savvy Diabetic

A Survival Guide

*Tips, Tools, and Techniques to Stay in
Control and Balance*

Joanne Laufer Milo

3DogArt Press
Corona Del Mar, CA

Published in the United States by 3DogArt Press, a division of 3DogArt.

ISBN-10: 09896385-0-2

Editor: Christy Jones, www.3DogArtPress.com

Layout and Design: Ray Sanford, www.SanfordWebSystems.com

Cover Design by Ryan McCoy, www.fewtr.com

Cover Art by Rebecca Stringer Korpita

"Dancing a Fine Line with Diabetes" original artwork, reprinted with permission from the artist, Rebecca Stringer Korpita, http://www.etsy.com/shop/korpita. Ms. Korpita is "an artist from the Mississippi Gulf Coast who loves color and humor. Her subject matter includes coastal life, the beach, southern culture, women, and pets and the people they own."

Additional artwork:

"Garden of Children" original artwork, reprinted with permission from the artist, Jody Bergsma, Bergsma Gallery Press, www.Bergsma.com

Broom Hilda comic strips by Russell Myers:

"BAW! HO HO HO..." 7/11/197? (year uncertain) "Oh, drat..." April 26, 1976 Copyright Tribune Media Services, Inc. All Rights Reserved. Reprinted with permission

Cartoons by John Chase, reprinted with permission from the artist, John Chase, www.chasetoons.com

Cartoons by Randy Glasbergen, reprinted with permission from the artist, Randy Glasbergen, www.glasbergen.com

Cartoons by Noah Fordyce, reprinted with permission from the artist, all rights reserved

For Richard

My hero, my savior, my consigliore,

my moral compass, my problem solver,

my medical consultant, my technology guru,

my chef and morning coffee brewer,

my raging humorist,

my best friend, my everything.

With all my appreciation and my love, always.

TABLE OF CONTENTS

Part 1: Living with Diabetes 3

1.1 ~ My Journey with Diabetes 5

Then it happened. No, I mean it really happened! 9

1.2 ~ The Basics about Diabetes... 11

In the United States 11

Worldwide... 12

1.3 ~ A Primer on Diabetes 13

Sugar, insulin and receptors—A simple explanation 13

What happens when you eat? 15

What happens in diabetes? 16

What do good and bad blood glucose levels mean? 17

1.4 ~ Control.. 19

Clinical control 20

Social control.. 22

Here are some real-life "what ifs": 22

Who is in control of your diabetes? 23

Who is in control of your environment?... 23

Part 2: The Essentials 25

2.1 ~ Basic Steps to Survival 27

Steps to surviving the system 27

Make lists..27

Resources to help you make your lists 28

Store your lists.. 30

Ask Questions 30

Buzzwords 31

2.2 ~ Control and Juggling **33**

    Control 33

    Juggling 34

    More juggling! 35

2.3 ~ Advocates and Support **37**

    Communicate your concerns and needs 38

    Ask questions and get answers 40

    Your support team 42

    Choosing an advocate 42

    Train your advocate to be successful 44

Part 3: Day to Day, 24/7 ....**47**

3.1 ~ Choosing Your Medical Team **49**

    How to choose your doctors 51

    Interviewing your doctor 53

    Questions to Ask Potential Endocrinologists / Healthcare Providers * 53

    Other resources to help you find a great doctor 54

3.2 ~ Hypoglycemia, Hyperglycemia and Unawareness **56**

3.3 ~ Time: How much time does it take to have diabetes? **61**

    Testing 62

    Changing needles or changing infusion sets, and taking insulin 62

    Going to your doctor/healthcare provider 62

    Getting lab work done 63

    Going to the pharmacy to get your supplies 63

    Treating hypoglycemia (low blood glucose) 63

    Treating hyperglycemia (high blood glucose) 63

    Following up on insurance claims and filling out forms 64

    Analyzing results 64

    Food, eating, and insulin 64

    Miscellaneous other stuff 65

3.4 ~ Your Medical Information **69**

3.5 ~ Visits to the Doctor, the Lab and Radiology **73**

Appointment with Your Doctor *74*

Trip to the lab *75*

Visit to Radiology: X-rays, CT scans and MRIs *76*

3.6 ~ Natural Disasters: Earthquakes, Tornadoes, Hurricanes and Floods *79*

Part 4: The Hospital vs. You **81**

4.1 ~ Hospital Management 101 .... **83**

4.2 ~ The LIST: What to Bring with You **89**

4.3 ~ Emergency Room — the ER **91**

4.4.~ Your Hospital Stay **95**

Here's your chance to establish yourself either you and/or your advocate. 96

4.5 ~ What about your Insulin Pump, CGMS, Syringes and Meters? **99**

Syringes, Insulin and Meters *101*

It's Mine! Give it a label *101*

4.6 ~ Hospital Food: You Are What You Eat **105**

Part 5: Travel Near and Far **107**

5.1 ~ Around Town and Short Trips **109**

Snacks and Glucose *111*

Some Suggested Sources of Quick Sugar *111*

Keep your Up-To-Date Lists with you *112*

Insulin Pumps, Rx's and Meters, Away from Home *112*

Eyeglasses: Back Up Pair and Rx *114*

Need a doctor on the road? *114*

5.2 ~ Faraway Journeys **117**

Security Check Points and TSA rules *117*

Carry a travel letter from your doctor, and labels for supplies and meds *120*

Carry-on vs. checked bags *120*

Pack snacks and low blood glucose treats or glucose tabs *121*

Chargers and power adapters *121*
Back-up supplies *121*
Back to Basics — your list *122*
Conversions *122*

Part 6: Lifestyle Issues **127**

6.1 ~ Having Babies or Not? **129**

6.2 ~ Spouses, Partners, Families and Friends **139**
A Diabetic Child in the Family *139*
A Young Adult with Diabetes *140*
Spouses and Partners *142*
How to Communicate *144*
Reach out to Resources *145*

Part 7: Coping Toolbox **147**

7.1 ~ Anger, Fear, Gratitude and More **149**

7.2 ~ How to Talk to a Diabetic **155**
What to Say: Do's and Don'ts *155*

7.3 ~ A Place to Vent **159**

7.4 ~ Laughter is the Best Medicine **163**
Fun with quotes *165*
Fun with Dr. Seuss* *166*
Fun with Cartoons *167*
Fun with Jokes *168*

7.5 ~ Giving Back **169**

Part 8: Final Words..**171**

   8.1 ~ Top Ten List.. 173

   8.2 ~ What's Next?... 175

   8.3 ~ Appreciations 177

   8.4 ~ In Remembrance 181

   8.5 ~ About the Author 183

Part 9: Appendix...**185**

   9.1 ~ Resources & References....................................... 187

      Research and Fund Raising Organizations.......................*187*

      Medical Supplies, Pumps and CGMS.............................*188*

      Technology and Website Resources *188*

      Wearable Medical ID and Products *189*

      Great Websites and Blogs *190*

   9.2 ~ Glossary **191**

   9.3 ~ Sample Medical Information Lists **197**

      My Sample Medical Information Sheet...........................*197*

      My Sample Schedule of Medications *198*

      My Sample Emergency Contact Sheet *199*

      Blank Form: My Medicine List **201**

      Blank Form and Wallet Card: MedicAlert Foundation **202**

   9.4 ~ Sample Hospital Diet Plans and Menus **203**

   9.5 ~ TSA Information for Travelers, 2013 ....**205**

   9.6 ~ Foreign Language Translations **209**

   9.7 ~ Conversion Charts **213**

What people are saying about *The Savvy Diabetic: TheA Survival Guide*

"The Savvy Diabetic: A Survival Guide is truly a survival guide on so many day-to-day issues that people with diabetes have to deal with 24/7. Joanne shares her life-long experiences in a very easy to read manner that combines knowledge, humor, practicality and humility. A must read for all of us folks living with diabetes and our close friends and family. I loved it!"

~ Steven Edelman MD, Professor of Medicine
University of California San Diego Veterans Affairs Medical Center
Founder and Director — Taking Control of Your Diabetes 501(c)3 http://www.tcoyd.org

"The Savvy Diabetic: A Survival Guide is terrific! You provide an incredible resource for anyone and everyone touched by type 1 diabetes. I was particularly touched by the anecdotes from people affected by the disease. Their stories reminded me that T1D isn't just about statistics or data or medical facts. It's about loved ones who deal with diabetes constantly. It's about how they come to grips with the reality that there is no break, no vacation, no moment away from thinking about it. It's 24/7; it's always "there". While those of us who don't have T1D but are part of the extended family will never be able to understand this in the same way as those with T1D do, your book gave me a glimpse into — and a deeper appreciation for — their world. That gift alone makes *The Savvy Diabetic: A Survival Guide* worth reading. Thank you for writing it."

~ Dick Allen, Grandfather of a 15-year old with type 1 diabetes
Chairman of the Board of Directors, JDRF International
Strategic Advisor, *Mary and Dick Allen Diabetes Center,*
Hoag Hospital, Newport Beach, CA

"Thriving with diabetes is a whole lot easier when you have a good doctor on your side and can understand and master our crazy medical system. But how can you ever make that happen? Joanne Milo has written a practical, humorous, straight-from-the-heart guidebook that provides the tips you need. *The Savvy Diabetic: A Survival Guide* is chock full of helpful hints to help you prepare for and handle hospitals, doctor visits, travel and everyday life with diabetes. Read it now!"

~ William H. Polonsky, PhD, CDE
Chief Executive Officer, Behavioral Diabetes Institute
Associate Clinical Professor, University of California, San Diego
whp@behavioraldiabetes.org

"Having written six books benefitting people with diabetes, I can honestly say that *The Savvy Diabetic: A Survival Guide* is the most user-friendly book about diabetes I have ever seen. The information is excellent and the organization, graphics, and quotes make it a pleasure to read. If you have diabetes, get this book!"

~ Gloria Loring
Singer, actress, and author
Coincidence Is God's Way of Remaining Anonymous
Parenting a Child with Diabetes

"In the complex journey of living with diabetes the most critical element is to find a guide. In addition to the people in your lives — your family and friends and health care providers — the best guide is someone in whose shoes you can walk. Joanne Milo is just that person. Her template for living with success, and facing the myriad challenges, will enable you to go on your journey with diabetes with the information and insights that you need, so you can be who you want to be and live how you want to live while managing your diabetes. Read her words, hear her voice, and follow her spirit — then hopefully you can dream every dream…"

~ Francine R. Kaufman, M.D.
Medtronic Diabetes Chief Medical Officer and Vice President,
Global Medical, Clinical and Health Affairs
Emeritus Professor of Pediatrics and Communications at USC
The Center for Diabetes, Endocrinology and Metabolism
Children's Hospital Los Angeles

"A breezy, light-hearted, down-to-earth book of do's and don'ts that spirits you through EVERYTHING about living with diabetes. It humorously captures the Zen-like constant awareness diabetes requires, let alone the over 8 hours weekly of direct management (who knew?). Each chapter has opening and closing summaries with great quotes, and bullet points make for an easy read and easy reference. The style and tone are just right — a must read for family and friends; they may not believe your life with diabetes otherwise! This book is like having a savvy friend with diabetes at your side."

~ Daniel Einhorn, MD, FACP, FACE
President, American College of Endocrinology
Medical Director, Scripps Whittier Diabetes Institute
Clinical Professor of Medicine, UCSD
President, Diabetes and Endocrine Associates, La Jolla, CA

"Excellent! Easy to read and so informative. Bottom line… provides knowledge which is powerful and will result in control. Thanks for the opportunity to be a more savvy nurse!"

~ Robyn Nelson, PhD, RN
Dean, College of Nursing, West Coast University, Irvine, CA

The Savvy Diabetic: A Survival Guide is a worthwhile book for the many diabetics like you. Successfully diabetes self-management takes science, commitment, and art. I can sense your struggle and joy in your journey. Now you have become an elder in the diabetes community and you are ready to share your experience and advice. Your book is screaming, "do what I say, but don't do what I did."

~ Dr. Ping H. Wang, MD
Professor and Director, Center for Diabetes Research and Treatment
Sue & Bill Gross Stem Cell Research Center, University of California, Irvine

"Joanne, I can see a lot of hard work and "heart" has gone into writing your story. We are increasingly using the "Voice of the Patient" in building new approaches to care and management of diabetes. *The Savvy Diabetic: A Survival Guide* brings that perspective front and center. The practical tips are wise and useful for many chronic illnesses, not just diabetes, such as storing your critical medical information on a flash drive to carry with you. Thanks for sharing the book."

~ Athena Philis-Tsimikas, MD
Executive Director and Chief Medical Officer
Scripps Whittier Diabetes Institute, La Jolla, CA
Associate Clinical Professor, Division of Diabetes and Endocrinology
University of California, San Diego, La Jolla, CA

"In *The Savvy Diabetic: A Survival Guide*, Joanne Milo lays out the steps and insights for a successful life with diabetes. Her chapters cover it all from diagnosis to venting in this great resource! Keep it on your bookshelf — different chapters will be handy on different days and in different years."

~ John Walsh, PA, CDTC
Author, speaker, clinician, and co-author of *Pumping Insulin*

Preface and Overview

"I wish I didn't have diabetes."
~Anna R., age 7, Type 1 diabetes since she was 4
and could not even pronounce the word diabetes.

As of early 2013, I've had Type 1 diabetes for just over 48 years (that's over 17,545 days and over 138,700 shots, plus infusion sites and CGMS sensors and finger sticks and over 100,000 meals and snacks). That's a whole lot of poking and jabbing and juggling and balancing.

Being a diabetic is a 24/7 deal. It never takes a vacation. But just saying 24/7 doesn't even begin to convey the constant nature of this disease.

It is truly 24 hours a day, every hour, 7 days a week, every day, minute by minute. I am continually monitoring:

➢ How I am feeling,

➢ How much or if my blood glucose is rising or falling,

➢ When and what I am eating or going to eat,

➢ When and how intensely I am exercising,

➢ How stressed I am,

➢ My blood glucose level if I am going to be driving or if I am having a sick day.

Having diabetes is omnipresent, ever changing and requires relentless vigilance. Then there is the more time needed for:

➢ Ordering prescriptions and supplies,

➢ Making and going to doctors' appointments,

➢ Handling interminable calls to correct insurance issues.

Plus there is the attention required to interact with:

> ➤ Family members,
> ➤ Friends,
> ➤ Co-workers and bosses and customers.

Some days are easier, some are harder, and some are downright impossible. Control is a big word in our world, as are carbs, blood glucose management, HbA1c, pumps, and CGMS. Definitions and more to come later in this book.

Far from being the "perfect" diabetic, I'm doing okay and I am surviving and living my life. And I've learned a lot from every experience. I hope some of my insights will help you to:

> ➤ Live well and in balance with diabetes,
> ➤ Survive the medical system as a diabetic,
> ➤ Feel validated in your emotions and feelings,
> ➤ Support someone who has diabetes,
> ➤ Provide medical care for someone with diabetes.

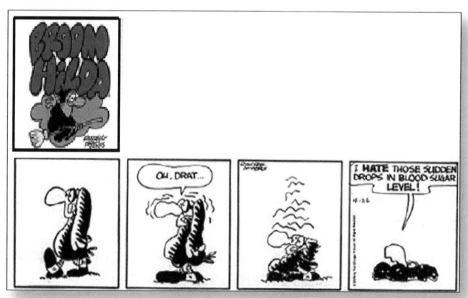

This is one of my favorite cartoons by Russell Myers, who kindly found this in his archives (from April 26, 1976) and gave me permission to share with you.

What lies ahead in this book

Going forward, you will find helpful planning and communication tips, tools, and techniques to juggle situations that make you feel out of control. This is a compilation of my experiences as well as input from an amazing group of friends with diabetes (and their spouses and friends) as well as wonderful blogs and bulletin boards to learn just what works (or doesn't work) when faced with hospitalization, laboratories, doctors' offices, travel, pregnancy, and other life surprises.

These tools to help you plan and survive the system as a diabetic include:

> Worksheets to keep your history, your medication and your schedule of how you take your meds,

> Tools for choosing the best doctors for you,

> Suggestions on how to:

⬦ interact with doctors' office staff,

⬦ interact with laboratory personnel and x-ray/imaging technicians,

⬦ get the most from your hospital staff (nurses, dieticians, doctors),

⬦ manage your insulin pump and CGMS in the hospital,

> What you'll need during a hospital stay,

> Travel tips,

> Thoughts about pregnancy and babies,

> Ideas about support and relationships and coping,

> A place set aside for venting your feelings.

If you are new to diabetes (or trying to understand it to be a better advocate to someone you care about), check out Chapter 1.3: A Primer on Diabetes. If you are a pro (medical or long timer with diabetes) you might just want to skip through that.

As you read, you'll find:

> *Stories of real diabetics and their real life experiences*

**SPECIFICS ON
"WHY THIS IS IMPORTANT AND
WHAT IF I DON'T?"**

TIP | Really good or special tip or point of discussion

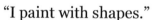

"I paint with shapes."
~ Alexander Calder, American sculptor, originator of the mobile

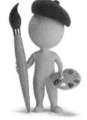

I hope this book is helpful to you. If you have additional tips or techniques, drop me a line at joanne@thesavvydiabetic.com or a post on www.facebook.com/TheSavvyDiabetic. I'd love to include them to my next edition.

Here's to staying healthy, successful and in control.

DISCLAIMER #1: I use the word, "diabetic," throughout this book to describe "persons with diabetes."

When I was first diagnosed, in 1965, my disease was called "diabetes mellitus" and I was referred to as a "diabetic." Then, in the early 1970s, my disease was renamed "juvenile diabetes," but I was still referred to as a "diabetic" or "juvenile diabetic."

About that time, discussions were surfacing on the issue of sensitivity to being labeled "diabetic." Patients felt it important to say they were "persons with diabetes" as diabetes doesn't define them. "I have "diabetes" but I am not a "diabetic.

And now, in the twenty first century, we are referred to as "Type 1 diabetics" or "T1D's", or "persons with Type 1 diabetes", which are not to be confused with Type 2 or Type 1.5 diabetics, even though we all have diabetes.

I am aware that the American Diabetes Association has made it a point to not use the word "diabetic", as a noun, so as not to give a "label" to those with the disease, diabetes.

According to the Merriam-Webster Dictionary, a "diabetic" is defined as "a person affected with diabetes.

I choose to use the term "diabetic" to refer to any "person with diabetes". This is not meant as a slight or insult but simply a shortcut. I do not mean to offend or upset those persons living with diabetes and I do understand the issue.

∾

"I yam what I yam, and that's all what I yam."
~ Popeye, the Sailor Man, cartoon fictional character

∾

I do know that diabetes does not define you, or any of us living with diabetes. Please read on, so you may learn some helpful tips, tools, and techniques for living your life as "persons with diabetes".

DISCLAIMER #2: The information contained within these pages should not be considered medical advice. You and your healthcare providers are responsible for any decisions made about your care and, therefore, you should work with them on your condition.

DISCLAIMER #3: Some of my comments about using your insulin pump, blood glucose meter, and CGMS in the hospital setting relate to my personal experiences and triumphs using my diabetes technology as an in-patient with full consent and cooperation of my attending physicians.

There is conflicting literature about whether pumps are safe to be used in an operating room environment. Some guidelines and manufacturers recommend removal for safety reasons in this environment. Although CGMS can be wonderful for ongoing monitoring of blood glucose, there are still no uniform approvals and definitive research demonstrating effectiveness in a hospital environment. Most hospitals have their own policies that require their staff to check blood glucose using approved hospital devices, even if a patient is using their own blood glucose meter or CGMS during the hospital stay. This doesn't mean that a hospital will not allow a patient to use their device but just that they will be accountable for using the approved standards for documentation and treatment.

Given this medical system mumbo jumbo, my best advice here is to discuss use of your own blood glucose meter, CGMS and insulin pump with your doctor or the attending healthcare providers, so that everyone involved with your hospitalization will be in agreement. It is particularly important to chat with your anesthesiologist about your devices prior to surgery. Every anesthesiologist who I worked with actually kept the CGMS receiver in his or her pocket and loved monitoring the information (current blood glucose and trending) during my surgical procedures.

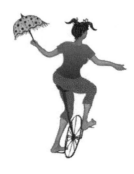

The Savvy Diabetic

A Survival Guide

PART 1: LIVING WITH DIABETES

1.1   My Journey with Diabetes

1.2   Diabetes Statistics, U.S. and Worldwide

⟡ In the United States

⟡ Worldwide

1.3   A Primer on Diabetes

⟡ Sugar, Insulin and Receptors

⟡ What happens when you eat?

⟡ What happens in diabetes?

⟡ What do good and bad blood glucose levels mean?

1.4   Control

⟡ Clinical control

⟡ Social control

⟡ Who's in control of your diabetes?

⟡ Who's in control of your environment?

1.1 ~ My Journey with Diabetes

"Step with care and great tact.
And remember that life's a great balancing act."
Dr. Seuss, American writer, poet and cartoonist

In the winter of 1965, I was just 11 years old and feeling so sick I could not make it to school. On a cold Monday in January, my pediatrician sat with Mom and me after hours, in his dark office, to teach us about my diagnosis. I had Type 1 diabetes (at the time, called diabetes mellitus).

I was terrified. I didn't feel well. Mom was crying, and I thought I was going to die from a disease that I didn't understand. The doctor taught Mom how to give me insulin injections, how to test the levels of sugar in my urine, and what foods I could no longer eat. Then he sent us home, for a scary first night as a diabetic.

I remember that first night at home as if it were yesterday. My mom gave me shots, had me pee on TesTape, give me chicken broth and pickles (for salt, as I had high ketones, I guess) and more shots. It was a very long, first night with diabetes.

That was the beginning of the next 48 years of living with, battling with, wrangling with, struggling with, coping with, and simply surviving with Type 1 diabetes. I immediately started on insulin injections, initially administered by Dad, an engineer but secretly a wannabe surgeon. He was outstanding at giving painless shots. But, given the psychological thinking of the time, the doctor thought it was "unwise" for a father (i.e., a male) to give injections to a pre-pubescent daughter. So Dad sadly turned over the shot tasks to Mom.

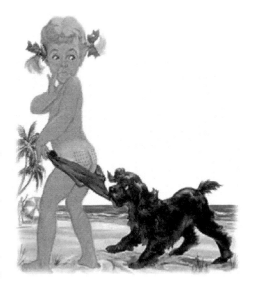

Mom was a nervous wreck. She would jab me with the syringe, she thought she "met resistance", she would stop, she would pull the syringe out and she would go back to step #1. This "poke and pull out" could go on for five to ten times per shot. It's surprising that I didn't spring a leak, as seen on the Zerex TV commercials that ran in the 1960's (in which a can of engine coolant was punctured and coolant sprayed out until the Zerex was added. The voiceover told us that Zerex Super Sealer stops cooling system leaks fast). I would tell Mom that I needed to add a can of Zerex and watch her cringe with sadness and maternal angst.

Not only that, but Mom was advised not to inject in the same place every day. So she developed a graphing system, on my buttocks using red mercurochrome dots in a five x five grid pattern, spaced one inch apart. On my first visit back to my pediatrician, he noticed the odd, geometric bright red rash on my behind and was puzzled. Mom explained her system to the doctor with great precision. Imagine how embarrassing the discussion of my buttocks was for me as an 11 year-old?

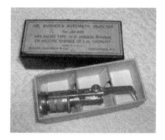

I rapidly learned to give myself my own injections of insulin, using the Busher Automatic Injector, a contraption that held the syringe and would automatically inject when you pushed a little lever.

I learned to test my urine for sugar with TesTape (a yellow strip of tape that turned varying shades of green to indicate how much was spilling into my urine). The amount of sugar in my urine would then determine how much insulin I needed before each meal.

Within a year, there was a new product for testing how much sugar I was spilling into my urine — CliniTest, which made me feel a bit like a mad scientist. First I had to discard my first pee, drink some water and wait until I could collect my second pee. Then, using an eye dropper, I would squeeze 10 drops of water plus five drops of urine into a test tube, add a fizzing tablet, wait 30 seconds, and

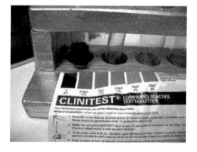

then compare the color to a chart posted on our bathroom wall. The results were not terribly accurate or definitive (2% or more could mean blood glucose of 200 or blood glucose of 500). But it was the best that was available at the time.

Even a 13 year old could quickly get the "right" answer by adding a few more drops of water and a few less drops of urine. Voila, my glucose readings were lower, in the good range. Who was I really fooling? But I just wanted to get good numbers and be normal.

My teenage years raged in, with all the usual emotions and the usual hormones in puberty. In high school, I had to deal with all the normal adolescent pressures of trying to fit in, dealing with hormones, school work, and family life all while trying to control my diabetes.

Around 1970, my parents bought me one of the first blood glucose monitor systems: the Ames Eyetone Reflectance Meter (which I've since donated to the FDA for its display of early technology). It was big and clunky, weighed about three pounds, plugged into the wall, cost $400 (that would be $2400 in today's money), and was analog rather than digital, like today's meters. But it provided a more accurate reading than

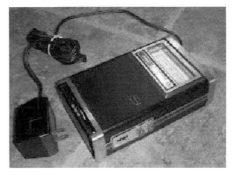

urine testing. And I was so fortunate that my parents could afford the expense. I also started with MDI (multiple daily injections) and found I managed my diabetes a little bit better.

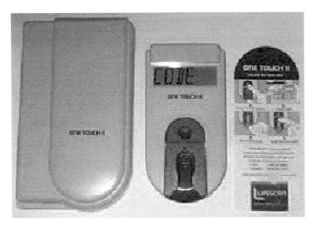

I entered college in 1972 and continued to use blood glucose meters. They were becoming smaller, faster and more accurate. I did my best to control, learning about living with roommates, managing the stress of midterms and finals, going to social and school activities, maintaining my exercise routine, my diabetes while living away from home and trying to figure out my life's direction.

By the 1980s, newer technologies had improved tools to assist in living with diabetes. HbA1c or Hemoglobin A1c (a laboratory test) was used to determine the average blood sugars over a 90 day span. More accurate meters, with quicker result times that were also more portable and less expensive (down to about $75) gave me more reliable results. Newer human insulin gave me better and faster absorption and purer quality.

Then in 2004, I started to use an insulin pump. Mine was an aqua blue Deltec Cozmo, which looked very cool and allowed me to make instantaneous insulin corrections to adjust to changes in my life, exercise, and diet.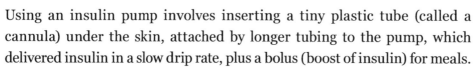

Using an insulin pump involves inserting a tiny plastic tube (called a cannula) under the skin, attached by longer tubing to the pump, which delivered insulin in a slow drip rate, plus a bolus (boost of insulin) for meals. What an amazing breakthrough for improving and allowing more freedom for diabetics.

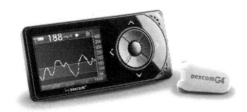 More recently, 2008 brought the continuous glucose monitoring system (CGMS) which involves placing a small (about ¾") sensor under the skin attached to a small transmitter. This sends a reading that indicates a blood glucose level, every five minutes to a read out receiver, which I carry in my pocket (or if my clothes do not have pockets, stuffed in my bra). I am able to track blood sugar changes constantly and instantly.

While current GGMS are not 100% accurate, I can see changes, and most importantly, respond to rising or to dropping trends in my blood glucose. The CGMS also provides audible and vibration alarms when the detected blood glucose levels go above or below my selected warning thresholds. Many are the nights when a CGMS buzzing alarm awakens me(or my husband) to warn me that my blood glucose is getting too high or too low. All of this technology is not a cure for diabetes. But the tools make it easier for me to maintain better control, given all the variables I juggle every day.

So, is this a happy ending to my story? Well, not yet. In the back of my mind, I have always aware that I could end up in the hospital (even for something non-diabetes related) or travel somewhere where foods are hard to calculate and activities and schedules are not part of my regular routine. Then all my control would be out of my control!

Then it happened. No, I mean it really happened!

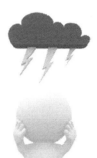

On the 4th of July weekend, 2008, I flew from California to Long Island, NY, to help my elderly mom move closer to us on the West Coast. We were at day two of our seven day trip to completely pack and move her. It was a dark and stormy night when we arrived back to our hotel room after dinner. I started to develop abdominal pains and I decided to call my doctor friend in California, who said, "Sounds like appendicitis, go to the ER."

Couldn't be!

Not liking his advice, I decided to get a second opinion. I called my internist's after hours exchange and requested the doctor call me in NY.

My husband looked at me and asked where my medication list was. I didn't have it. He asked me where my list of doctors and emergency contacts was. I didn't have that either. I only planned on being in New York for seven days and hadn't planned on getting sick! My husband pulled out his laptop and began quickly transcribing my critical information, allergies, medications and medical contacts, in case I might not be able to provide that information from memory later.

My internists returned my call shortly, and after a few questions said, "Sounds like appendicitis, go to the ER." I asked if it could wait until I returned to California. He said, "No." When I asked if I could wait until the morning to see if I felt better, he said, "No! Go to the ER immediately." I was now officially out of options for escaping the trip to the hospital!

On the way out, we stopped at the hotel's business office just long enough to print out the medications and doctors' lists and headed to the ER.

I didn't have time for this. But mostly I was not prepared. I hadn't planned on being hospitalized, I didn't have all my medical information, and now I was faced with all new doctors. And I was scared. I had avoided ever being in the hospital and now, I was heading to the emergency room in the hospital, without my regular doctors, in pain, facing surgery, and an undetermined hospital stay.

My education on being a diabetic in a hospital began that night. Suddenly I was out of control, needing to communicate my medications, my diet, my other health issues, facing anesthesia and establishing a relationship with new doctors. All I could do was scramble to get my information together and navigate a new hospital environment in an unfamiliar city with impending surgery. And I was in pain and didn't feel very well.

Being back in my home town, I started calling childhood friends at 7:00 AM for a referral to a surgeon and, by 8:00 AM I had connected to a great team of surgeons. My surgery was scheduled for 3:00 PM that day, and I was out of the hospital by 1:00 PM the following day.

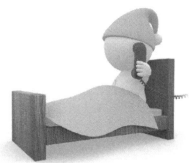

I survived.

Since then, I have been hospitalized three more times (also not related to diabetes) and, additionally, have had several outpatient surgeries. Each time, I learned more about what I needed to survive the medical system, as a savvy diabetic.

What I hope to share with you are tips, tools, and techniques that will help you gain a new level of control over your life with diabetes, along with an increased sense of psychological mastery.

"The need to write comes from the need to
make sense of one's life and discover one's usefulness."
~ John Cheever, American novelist and short story writer

1.2 ~ The Basics about Diabetes

"I plan on living forever.
So far, so good."

~ Steven Wright, American comedian, actor and writer

BASIC: n. bāsik: *The essential facts or principles of a subject or skill*

According to the National Institutes of Health, there are 4 types of diabetes: Type 1, Type 2, Type 1.5 and Gestational.

In the United States

- ➢ 25.8 million children and adults in the U.S. have diabetes or around 8.3% of the U.S. population. Stated differently, on average about one out of 12 people you meet has some form of diabetes.
- ➢ Of those with diabetes, 18.8 million have been diagnosed, and 7.0 million are still undiagnosed.
- ➢ 1.9 million new cases of diabetes are diagnosed in people over age 20 each year, which works out to a new case of diabetes being diagnosed <u>every 30 seconds</u>.

Regarding Type 1 diabetes (T1D) in the United States:*

- ➢ It affects approximately 5% of the total diabetic population, or around 1.3 million Americans.
- ➢ Each year, more than 15,000 children and 15,000 adults (around 80 people per day) are diagnosed with Type 1 diabetes.
- ➢ 85% of Type 1 diabetics living in the US are over the age of 20.

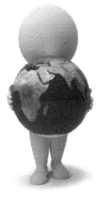

Worldwide

- ➤ Worldwide, there is an estimated 375 million people, corresponding to 6.4% of the world's adult population, living with diabetes. (World Health Organization)
- ➤ The total number of living diabetics has doubled since 1980, and is expected to grow to 552 million by 2030, corresponding to 7.8% of the adult population, (American Diabetes Association).
- ➤ The rate of Type 1 diabetes incidence among children under the age of 14 is estimated to increase by 3% annually worldwide (American Diabetes Association).

With this enormous and ever-increasing number of diabetics, you might think that, in general, all healthcare professionals and institutions are quite skilled at caring for patients with diabetes. Sadly, this is not true.

Unfortunately, the medical system is neither prepared nor adequately educated to provide services for the burgeoning number of newly diagnosed diabetes cases nor the wide range of individual particular diabetics needs, especially in hospitals or labs.

The problem is particularly acute for Type 1 diabetics, who represent a minority 5% of all diabetics. With only 1.3 million Type 1 diabetics in the U.S., many health care systems simply do not know what the standard of care applicable to Type 1 diabetes or how to handle those individuals in their facilities. They tend to treat Type 1 diabetics the same as Type 2 diabetics, which can easily put Type 1 diabetics at risk.

What can you do to increase your chances of surviving healthfully in this quagmire? Keep reading to find tips, tools, and techniques to help you get prepared and smoothly navigate successfully, as a person with any type of diabetes.

1.3 ~ A Primer on Diabetes

"If you've heard this story before, don't stop me,
because I'd like to hear it again."
~Groucho Marx, American comedian, actor and singer

For those of you who are new to diabetes, below is a short description of how sugar and insulin work in the human body. It is not a technically detailed and rigorous discussion of cellular metabolism and endocrine functions, but is meant to provide a novice with a simple description of diabetes to have a basic understanding of the factors and terms covered in this book. If you are technically savvy, then you'll understand that I'm trying not to make things more complicated than a novice needs to know, and you may want to skip over this section.

Sugar, insulin and receptors — A simple explanation

All of the living cells in the body burn oxygen and nutrients to live, and give up carbon dioxide, heat and waste in return. They get their food and oxygen from the blood stream. The favorite fuel at the cellular level is glucose (a form of sugar) that can be absorbed into the cell from the blood stream. To burn the sugar, the cells also need insulin.

Insulin is a hormone produced by the beta cells located in the pancreas. Beta cells basically lie around in the pancreas and when they sense an increase in blood glucose (blood sugar) levels, these react by secreting insulin. At that point, the blood stream contains both glucose and insulin along with oxygen necessary for cellular life.

The final key to the process is for the insulin receptors at the cellular level to let the insulin into the cell to burn the available glucose that was absorbed from the bloodstream. The body regulates the burn of fuel by juggling the amount of blood glucose and insulin along with turning insulin receptors on or off, all the while trying to keep you at the proper body temperature.

So far, glucose is fuel and you need insulin and oxygen to go with the fuel, and the insulin receptors let the insulin into the cell to allow the glucose to be burned. Sounds pretty easy, right?

Now, let's look at a typical 24-hour day, starting at bedtime. Many people fall into a deep sleep for several hours and may snore, breathe deeply, expend higher levels of sleep energy. Then, later in the sleep cycle, they may rest more peacefully, except for short periods of dreaming. When they wake in the morning, the body responds with enough extra energy to get up and going. Then there is breakfast, with or without morning exercise, and off to school or work. Work can be vigorous for some (for example, a construction worker) or alternately, sedentary for another (perhaps an accountant). On to lunch and then, the afternoon. After school/work, there can be play, chores, shopping, or exercise. Then dinner, relaxing, and back to bed.

Clearly, everybody is different. Even more clearly, everyone's need for fuel and energy is constantly changing throughout the day, and varying day to day.

➢ What if you run five miles on Sunday at 10 AM, but on Monday at 10 AM you are sitting in a meeting?

➢ What if you had to get up suddenly and chase after the dog?

➢ What if you were one of those superhuman people you read about who lifts a car off of a trapped baby stroller?

There is no fixed answer as to how much energy (glucose + insulin+ oxygen) your body will need until you are involved in that specific activity or action.

Your liver stores extra glucose in a form called glycogen. It can push glycogen into your blood stream when you need it. In fact, most people get their first morning pre-breakfast, pre-coffee boost of energy from some glycogen, courtesy of their liver. That increases the glucose in the blood stream, so the beta cells react by secreting insulin and the insulin receptors let the insulin into the cells. Therefore, when you wake up, you can make energy, which gets you out of bed.

What happens when you eat?

When you eat, food begins to be absorbed into your body though the mucous membranes, or if it is more complex, through the digestive tract. Foods are basically, proteins, fats or carbohydrates. And carbohydrates can be anything from simple sugars (which are absorbed without digestion) to complex whole grains and starches that take a long time be digested before they are absorbed. Some carbohydrates enter your blood stream almost immediately, such as refined sugar, orange juice, lactose (sugar) in milk, or jelly beans.

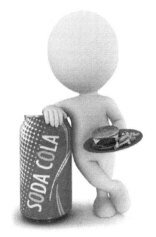

If you eat fast-acting (quickly absorbed) carbohydrates, you will cause your blood glucose level to spike. Normal beta cells will respond to the spike in blood glucose with a spike in insulin. You will be swamped with fuel and insulin and the body will start revving up. Later, when all the sugars are gone, the body stops producing insulin and the blood glucose stabilizes.

In fact, you may have produced a bit too much insulin and that will cause you to burn a bit too much blood glucose which will cause your blood glucose levels to fall below the desired steady state level. Low blood glucose can make you feel sleepy, or jittery, or have headaches, or be short tempered and hungry. This is the famous 10 AM "sugar crash" that kids get after eating a high carb breakfast. In fact, milk (lactose), corn flakes, bananas, and a spoonful of sugar are all individually fast-acting carbs that will cause the blood glucose level to spike. Add them all together and you have a potent recipe for two hours of wind-up followed by two hours of a not-so-nice crash.

What if you do eat too much fuel, and cause your body to make insulin, but the combination of blood glucose and insulin is more than you need to burn to keep alive and warm? Well, you could run around to burn it off. Or your body could heat up to burn it off, but since our body regulates our temperature, that doesn't happen. So your body does the only thing it can with the extra fuel and insulin. It stores it for later.

Where does it put it? Some of it is kept in the liver as glycogen. The rest is converted into fat, and stored for some day in the future when you might run out of food. Waste not, want not.

What happens in diabetes?

Now, for the diabetes part.

There are four main types of diabetes.

> ➤ In Type 1 diabetes, the insulin-producing beta cells in the pancreas are destroyed, and the body cannot produce the insulin necessary for sustain life. Type 1 diabetics currently must inject insulin or wear an insulin pump. This form was previously referred to as insulin-dependent diabetes mellitus (IDDM) or juvenile diabetes.

> ➤ Type 2 diabetes results from insulin resistance (a condition in which cells fail to use insulin properly), sometimes combined with an insulin deficiency. This form was previously referred to as non-insulin-dependent diabetes mellitus (NIDDM) or adult-onset diabetes.

> ➤ The third main form, gestational diabetes, occurs when pregnant women without a previous diagnosis of diabetes develop high blood glucose levels. It may, but not necessarily, precede development of type 2 diabetes, and requires very close blood glucose monitoring throughout the pregnancy to ensure delivery of a healthy baby.

> ➤ The newest type, often diagnosed in adults over 30, is Latent Autoimmune Diabetes in Adults (LADA), sometimes known as Type 1.5 diabetes. LADA is often misdiagnosed as Type 2 diabetes because of the age it is diagnosed. However, people with LADA do not have insulin resistance like those with Type 2 diabetes. LADA is characterized by age, a gradual increase in insulin necessity, positive antibodies, low C-peptide, lack of family history of Type 2 diabetes, and insulin resistance medications being ineffective. Treatment for LADA is the same as for Type 1 diabetes.

From the descriptions above, Type 1 diabetics and some Type 2 diabetics do not make any insulin, and therefore they must take insulin every day just to live. Some Type 2 diabetics do not make enough insulin so they must also supplement with insulin.

However, most Type 2 diabetics have a problem at the insulin receptor level. They experience high blood glucose or sometimes high insulin levels (or both) because the receptors won't let the insulin in and the cells can't burn the glucose.

In any case, the body's automatic response system is broken and unable to adjust:

➢ Insulin production,

➢ Blood glucose,

➢ Turning on and off insulin receptors,

➢ Food intake,

➢ Energy requirements,

➢ Body temperature.

To make things worse, many medications cause blood glucose to rise or fall, independent of insulin. It can be very common for glucose levels to rise (raising insulin demand) when the body's immune system is trying to fight off an infection, deal with an injury, or cope with high levels of emotional stress and anxiety.

What do good and bad blood glucose levels mean?

If you are a non-diabetic person, the body regulates blood glucose to around 100mg/dL. Depending on the time of day, your blood glucose might be as low as 80 mg/dL, following extreme exercise, or as high as 120 mg/dL while your body is trying to digest that very sweet desert you just ate while watching television. But pretty quickly, the blood glucose returns to normal.

If you are a Type 1, non-insulin producing diabetic, without insulin, your blood glucose will simply rise without limit to 200, then 300, then 400, then 500, etc. As the blood glucose gets higher and higher, you feel sicker and sicker. You can't think right, you can't see right, you can't coordinate right, your blood gets syrupy thick and your heart has to work harder to move your blood around. You might become very thirsty. Left unchecked, high blood glucose will lead to death, but it will take a while.

Some people get used to feeling "pepped up" with higher blood glucose, and due to the shortage of insulin to store the extra blood glucose as fat, Type 1 diabetics with higher blood glucose levels often do not gain weight. But there are complications that occur over time when blood glucose levels are too high, including blindness, kidney failure, heart disease, and sometimes amputation of extremities.

If you suddenly get too much insulin, your blood glucose will start dropping. You can't think right, you can't see right, you can't coordinate right, your blood gets thin. Often people with low blood glucose levels feel very jittery, and many become non-communicative or even combative. At very low blood glucose levels (below 40), people will begin to show signs of losing consciousness. By the time blood glucose levels drop below 30, people are in extreme danger of having convulsions or entering into a diabetic coma and dying.

So, if you start at a perfect 100 mg/dL and your blood glucose goes up by 80 points, you might feel a bit off or you might feel pretty good and frisky. Conversely, if you start at a perfect 100 mg/dL and your blood glucose drops by 80, you could be unconscious or in convulsions or nearing death.

For low blood glucose, you reduce insulin and add carbohydrates (either fast acting or slow acting) until your blood glucose gets back into a normal range. If you have high blood glucose, you avoid food and add some insulin to bring things back to normal. This food / insulin dance is called chasing. It is like trying to drive your car with your foot pressing on the brake while another person's foot is pressing the gas. Things can get very scary when both of you are pressing at the same time.

Now it can get even trickier

Let's say you see your blood glucose is too high (but unknown to you, it is already dropping back toward normal). So you add some insulin. The extra insulin makes the blood glucose drop even faster. The next thing you know, you are passing through the normal zone and heading into the low blood glucose zone. So you have to chase the dropping blood glucose by eating some fast acting carbs. Eventually you get your blood glucose back into the normal range, but the extra insulin and extra food were converted to fat. What a challenging balancing act, which can make you fat, adding insult to injury!

"When you reach the end of your rope,
tie a knot in it and hang on."
~ *Thomas Jefferson, American Founding Father*

1.4 ~ Control

"Don't take the bull by the horns, take him by the tail.
Then you can let go when you want to."
~ Josh Billings, American humorist and lecturer

No single word is more significant to a diabetic than control. It has so many times and ways a diabetic can find themselves "out of control". Is it a verb? Is it a noun? Is it a job position? Is it a circumstance?

CONTROL: [kuhn-trohl]

As a verb:

1. To exercise authoritative or dominating influence over; direct.

2. To adjust to a requirement; regulate: controlled trading on the stock market; controls the flow of water.

3. To hold in restraint; check: struggled to control my temper.

4. To reduce or prevent the spread of: control insects; controlled the fire by dousing it with water.

5. To verify or regulate (a scientific experiment) by conducting a parallel experiment or by comparing with another standard.

6. To verify (an account, for example) by using a duplicate register for comparison.

As a noun:

1. Authority or ability to manage or direct: lost control of the skidding car; the leaders in control of the country.

2. One that controls; a controlling agent, device, or organization.

3. An instrument or set of instruments used to operate, regulate, or guide a machine or vehicle.

4. A restraining device, measure, or limit; a curb: a control on prices.
   a. A standard of comparison for checking or verifying the results of an experiment.
   b. An individual or group used as a standard of comparison in a control experiment.

5. An intelligence agent who supervises or instructs another agent.

6. A spirit presumed to speak or act through a medium.

After 48 years of diabetes, I am beginning to think it is somehow linked to Noun #6, some spiritual force acting though a medium!

Clinical control

Clinical diabetic control relates to how well diabetics are able to regulate their average blood glucose (as tested by an HbA1c lab test) along with the range of high and low blood glucose levels they encounter on a daily basis. For diabetics with blood glucose ranging between 40 and 300, their average may be a reasonable 120 (5.6 HbA1c) but they are definitely bouncing all over the place and probably do not feel very well a lot of the time

So there is long term control of blood glucose (where are you on average), and there is short term control of blood glucose (where are you at the moment).

Some people have the concept that their doctor (hopefully an endocrinologist) is in control of the medical treatment. They are certainly in control of your medications and lab tests. But unless you are with them 24/7, they are much more like an air traffic controller hundreds of miles away in a control tower and not the actual pilot of your plane (i.e., your diabetic body).

So who is flying your plane? Assuming you are an adult, then you are the pilot. If you are an infant, a child or someone who needs assistance, then you are much more of a passenger and some adult or caregiver is trying to fly your plane for you. Once again, assuming you are the pilot of your own plane, you are in control. Or are you?

If your body and metabolism was completely predictable, then maybe you could add a little food, add a little insulin, add a little exercise and the blood glucose needle on the dash board (your glucose meter) would hover around 100 all day and night.

But the truth is (as we discuss later in the book) that the skies you fly in are anything but calm. There are up drafts and down drafts, and cloud banks and fog and sometimes even thunder and lightning and even moments of pitch blackness.

To make things even worse, sometimes when you add some throttle or try to steer around something, the plane (your body) simply ignores your best efforts and goes in some other direction completely. It is as if the plane's controls were not even connected to the wings or engines. There is that control word again.

Great! You are the pilot who is in control of the controls of a plane that has a mind of its own and is going out of control while flying though capricious weather.

But wait, what happens when you are asleep or worse yet, sick or unconscious and unable to fly the plane? If you have a trained and willing advocate (spouse or similar), then sometimes your copilot has to take control. But then you have to remember that your body is the plane, so it is very hard for a copilot to fly a plane when he or she is not actually in the plane. To your copilot, it is much more like flying one of those remote radio controlled planes, except as we stated earlier, the controls do not always work correctly. Hey, maybe the copilot calls the doctor in the remote control tower (you have to imagine the doctor actually answers the phone) and your copilot starts asking questions like "How do I land this thing?" But wait, when you or your copilot calls the control tower you get an automated message, "If this is an emergency, please call 911."

Social control

Another major control factor could be called social control. How do you minimize the impact of your diabetes treatment on your professional and social life?

> ➤ What if you are in an important business meeting with important clients and you suspect your blood glucose is dropping?
> ➤ Or maybe you are in the middle of a church wedding?
> ➤ Or maybe you are the bride?
> ➤ Or maybe you are on a first date?

Do you break away from the situation to test?

Here are some real-life "what ifs":

> ➤ What if you find you need food and soon, but the meal or breaks are not scheduled for some time?
> ➤ What if your flight is held on the ground for several hours causing takeoff and meal service to be delayed?
> ➤ What if you are under good control as you get up to give a presentation, but the adrenaline kicks in and your blood glucose starts to drop like a rock or skyrocket like a missile?
> ➤ What if you are at a play and your insulin pump detects a delivery failure and starts sending out an alarm?
> ➤ What if you tucked the insulin pump inside your bra so you could wear your best full length gown without having your pump clipped to your belt?
> ➤ What if your gown has a high neckline, so the only way to get to the bra is from the bottom?

Who is in control of your diabetes?

This is a significant question regarding you, your doctors and healthcare professionals, and emergencies.

- ➤ What factors of your diabetes treatment does your doctor control and dictate?
- ➤ Who is making the minute to minute decisions on blood glucose, food, insulin, exercise, medications, etc.?
  - ✧ Who is in control if you are unconscious and the paramedics are called?
  - ✧ Who sets the "rules" in the ER or a hospital?
  - ✧ What if your diabetes supplies are taken away or withheld from you?
  - ✧ What if the medical staff does not have or will not administer critical medications?
  - ✧ What if the doctor decides the nurses will measure your blood glucose and then decide your insulin dose? This can depend on whether you are conscious or unconscious or in the emergency room or a hospital bed.
  - ✧ Who manages your diabetes when you are unable?
  - ✧ Do you have a trained advocate with a Durable Power of Attorney (DPA) to act on your behalf?
  - ✧ Do you have a backup in case your DPA is your spouse and you are both involved in an accident together?

Who is in control of your environment?

This is another significant question that bears some attention.

- ➤ What if you are on vacation in Africa or Tibet or just plain old New Orleans and a Katrina-size hurricane, earthquake or tsunami arrives (no power, no food, no water, no refrigeration, no open pharmacies).
- ➤ What if you are traveling in some foreign country and they want to seize your diabetes supplies?
- ➤ What if your hotel room is robbed and your diabetes supplies are stolen?
- ➤ What if you just lose your glucose meter?
- ➤ What if your pump / infusion set stop working and your blood glucose starts rising?

What social situations do you need to manage or maneuver through? Who is in control of the social situation?

Bottom line, nothing is more sacred to a diabetic than his/her blood glucose meter and insulin delivery system (syringes or pumps). Just like in a Clint Eastwood movie, you don't touch his gun or his horse.

All of this puts the diabetic in the position of constantly being extremely aware of: controlling

➢ Insulin, meters and diabetes supplies,

➢ Blood glucose in the short run vs. food vs. insulin vs. exercise vs. stress vs. rest,

➢ Blood glucose in the long run,

➢ Trying to avoid other health problems and other diabetes-related complications,

➢ Effects of environmental factors,

➢ Healthcare professionals' advice and recommended medications,

➢ Social and business situations and their impact on diabetes treatment.

Don't forget, you have to do this in your sleep, too. No wonder we hear the word control, from the moment we are diagnosed and forever on.

"You'll get mixed up, of course, as you already know.
You'll get mixed up with many strange birds as you go.

So be sure when you step. Step with care and great tact
and remember that Life's a Great Balancing Act.

Just never forget to be dexterous and deft.
And never mix up your right foot with your left."

~ Dr. Seuss, American writer, poet and cartoonist

PART 2: THE ESSENTIALS

Basic Steps to Survival

- ✧ Steps to surviving the system
- ✧ Make lists
- ✧ Resources to help you make your lists
- ✧ Store your lists
- ✧ Ask questions
- ✧ Buzzwords

Control and Juggling

- ✧ Control
- ✧ Be prepared

Advocates and Support

- ✧ Communicate your concerns and needs
- ✧ Ask questions and get answers
- ✧ Your support team
- ✧ Choosing your advocates
- ✧ Train your advocate to be successful

2.1 ~ Basic Steps to Survival

"I am prepared for the worst, but hope for the best."
~ Benjamin Disraeli, British Prime Minister, literary figure

KEY TOPICS

- Be proactive, be prepared
- Lists
- Ask Questions, write down answers

Each type of diabetes is a distinct disease, although they do share certain symptoms and treatments. But it is critical to be treated properly for our type of diabetes. So what can we do to protect ourselves from the system and educate the medical professionals?

Steps to surviving the system

There are several steps we can take to ensure that we survive the system:

- ➤ Be proactive,
- ➤ Be prepared,
- ➤ Ask questions,
- ➤ Communicate,
- ➤ Be your own best advocate,
- ➤ Assume the doctors or nurses don't understand your diabetes.

You have diabetes and you know what you do to take care of yourself. The word *unexpected* literally means something you do not expect. But when you least expect it, the unexpected can happen. To be prepared, *expect the unexpected.*

Make lists

There is a lot to remember about you and your medications, such as:

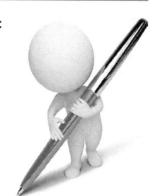

- ➤ Name (generic or brand),
- ➤ Dosage (the strength and unit of measure, such as 10 mg or 50 mcg),
- ➤ When you take them (twice a day, with meals, etc.),
- ➤ For what condition (diabetes, protect your kidneys, neuropathy, etc.),
- ➤ Any drug allergies and reactions (penicillin gives me a rash, etc.).

Then you have to remember details about your:

- ➤ Health insurance,
- ➤ Doctors and medical specialists,
- ➤ Driver's license,
- ➤ Emergency contacts.

If you make these lists and have them available to you, you will be better prepared to give accurate and useful information to the medical team taking care of you.

Specifically, these lists include:

- ➤ All your medications and supplements,
- ➤ Everything to which you have allergic reactions,
- ➤ Dosages (how much and when you take each),
- ➤ Detail the condition for what you take each medication (including whether it is critical or optional),
- ➤ Your doctors, their contact information, and specialty,
- ➤ Your insurance card(s) and driver's license,
- ➤ Significant members of your support system (spouse, children, friends) and their contact information,

➤ Your durable power of attorney for healthcare up to date,

➤ Items you will need if you are hospitalized,

➤ Items in an emergency pack of supplies. This is good for day trips or just in case.

Resources to help you make your lists

There are lots of ways to make your lists. In the appendix, section 9.3, you will find a variety of ways to lay out your medical information. I've included the lists that I use but there are many available online.

My Medicine List, a free link to a customizable form, is available via ASHP Research and Education Foundation, a philanthropic arm of the American Society of Health-System Pharmacists (www.ASHPFoundation.org, under the heading of Advancing Practice, My Medicine List). My Medicine List form is available also in the appendix, section 9.3.

Health Vault is a free site offered by Microsoft (www.healthvault.com), as a "safe, convenient place for managing your family's important health information," using Microsoft HealthVault to store data. There are tabs for medications, health conditions, allergies, insurance providers and emergency contacts. And you can add different profiles for family members. All you have to do is sign up and upload your information.

AARP Health Record, free to all AARP members (age 50 or over), uses the Microsoft HealthVault. You will need to:

➤ be a member of AARP (www.aarp.org and click on the JOIN button or 1-800-OUR-AARP or 1-800-687-2277) and,

➤ then open a free HealthVault account (www.healthvault.com).

Your information can be accessed by any internet connection, via smart phone or tablet. And you can decide you may have access to your information as well as store lab results and x-rays.

MedicAlert Foundation is a fee-based membership program which includes your medical information in a printable format, as well as an emergency wallet card and a free basic medical ID. You are assigned a MedicAlert ID number, which can be accessed anytime, from anywhere, via a toll-free number to a medically trained staff member, available 24/7, in case of an emergency. (www.medicalert.org).

Gazelle by Quest Diagnostics offers a free mobile app that allows you to see, store and share your vital health information, anytime and anywhere. You may receive your lab test results directly to your mobile device from Quest, as well as access your prescription medications and dosages, store you emergency and doctor contacts, allergies, and medical and immunization histories.

Store your lists

What do I do with this information? By the time this book is published, I'm sure there will be many more free options for storing your medical information. But I still recommend that you carry a hard copy of your information with you (in your purse or wallet) as well as on a USB drive and/or *in the cloud*.

Flash drives are cheap and small. Buy a 4 GB flash drive and store your data. Attach the drive to your keychain or insulin pump so you always have it with you.

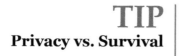

You can also keep copies of the information in the cloud (SkyDrive, DropBox, iCloud, etc.) but some healthcare settings cannot access that information.

TIP **Privacy vs. Survival**	What about the issue of keeping your medical information private? What if someone finds your information? This boils down to your personal feelings.

Here is the question to ask for yourself:

Would I rather risk the invasion of my privacy in order to make sure, in the event that I am unconscious or seriously ill or wounded, that the medical personnel treating me will have immediate access to my medical information?

For me, that answer is yes.

Ask Questions

It is easy to get flustered in a medical setting or when you are ill. Being prepared with your concerns ahead of time will help you get your questions answered and address important issues.

Bring a pen and paper to check off your questions and write the answers and jot down any follow up questions.

➢ Write down your concerns and questions before you see a medical professional.

➢ If you can, make a copy so he/she can read along.

There's a handy new device on the market by LiveScribe, called the SmartPen. This pen can record and synchronize what you're writing and what you're hearing as you take notes. You can record everything your doctor says and later replay any part of the consultation, along with your notes, for review. It is sold online at Amazon.com and on the Live Scribe website and costs between $100 and $250, depending on features.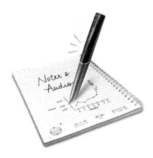

Buzzwords

As a preview of the next 2 chapters, the two big buzzwords you live with as a person with diabetes are:

➢ Control

➢ Advocacy

You most likely do your best to maintain control of all the variables that go into managing your medical issues. When that freedom is taken away due to hospitalization, you will need to advocate for your needs. You might need to ask a family member or friend to advocate for you, if you are too ill. With control and advocacy, you will insure the best possible outcome to survive your emergency or medical excursion so that you can get on with your life.

A QUICK REVIEW OF KEY TOPICS:
BASIC STEPS OF SURVIVAL

- Be proactive:
  - Be Prepared,
  - Expect the unexpected.
- Make lists of your medications, allergies, emergency contacts and medical team:
  - Use your own list or one of the many online services.
  - Keep a hard copy and the file stored on a flash drive or in the cloud.
- Ask questions, write down answers:
  - Bring paper and pen,
  - Write down the answers to your questions and any follow-up questions or issues.

2.2 ~ Control and Juggling

"If everything seems under control,
you're just not going fast enough."

~ *Mario Andretti, Italian-born American race car driver*

KEY TOPICS

- Control is important.
- Living with diabetes makes you a professional juggler.

Control

Here's the word we've heard since the first day we were diagnosed with diabetes. We discussed this in-depth in section 1.3. What's involved in control?

We must:

> Control our blood glucose levels,

> Control our stress levels,

> Control our insulin levels,

> Control our exercise levels,

> Control what we eat,

> Control our environment,

> Control our medical team,

> Control our attitude.

We do this to varying degrees of success from day to day, depending on variables in our lives, some of which we can control, most of which we can't.

There are plenty of resources to help you control and manage your diabetes on a day to day basis:

➤ doctors, certified diabetes educators and other medical professionals,

➤ family and friends,

➤ websites, blogs and online chats,

➤ books and lectures.

But, what about those routine or unexpected times, which are bound to come up and make our lives all the more challenging?

Juggling

Juggl-ing: n [jəgəl/' ing]

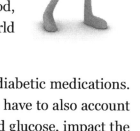

1. *Continuously tossing into the air and catching (a number of objects) so as to keep at least one in the air while handling the others*

2. *Coping with by adroitly balancing*

Adroitly? Give me a break! How adroitly can you balance your blood glucose, insulin, exercise, job, work and day-to-day stress?

Diabetes truly is a juggling act. You manage insulin, other meds, food, exercise, rest, stress (from family, work, health, co-workers, the world condition), and schedules, throughout the day, every day.

You have to take insulin (by injection or insulin pump) or oral anti-diabetic medications. But you have to determine how much to take throughout the day. You have to also account for other medications you need to take and how they affect your blood glucose, impact the absorption of your insulin and affect your appetite and energy levels.

Then there is food. Carb counting, or how many carbohydrates you plan to eat at any given time, helps you to calculate how much insulin you need for that food. You also have to factor in how much exercise (intensity, duration, and time of day) you've done or plan to do, how you are feeling (moods and illness) as well as the glycemic index (how readily absorbed the carbs will be) along with the overall balance of carbs, proteins, and fats.

There are so many questions and calculations you must do:

- ➤ Do you need to take less insulin, eat more food and what kind?
- ➤ You are supposed to do this for every food?
- ➤ What if your meal times vary?
- ➤ Or food isn't delivered when you expect it?
- ➤ What if there is more sugar content in the food, at a restaurant than you expected or accounted for?
- ➤ What if you are sticking to a diet?

More juggling!

What about stress? The impact of stress varies. It can either increase your blood glucose levels or decrease it. How are you supposed to know? What if you must deal with stress but can't change it or get rid of it?

Blood glucose testing provides you data either from a Continuous Glucose Monitoring Systems (CGMS) and/or a blood glucose meter. You are always checking to find out what your blood glucose is and what you need to do to correct or adjust.

This makes me tired just thinking about it, much less writing about it.

So you say, I'm tired of this so I'll just let it all do whatever but then you end up chasing and making insulin or food corrections later. You still face the possibility of coping with symptoms of low or high blood glucose, which can leave you feeling even more tired.

Quite the juggling act.

> *"I feel like I have to micro-manage my life."*
>
> Sue B., Type 1 diabetes for one year

A QUICK REVIEW OF KEY TOPICS:
CONTROL AND JUGGLING

- Control is essential and so important, but it can definitely be elusive.
- Juggling all the variables involved in managing diabetes is an important skill set.

Diabetes does not take a vacation. When your diabetes gets out of control, you don't feel well, and you may not be thinking clearly enough to make good decisions. You live with the fear of the consequences that take their toll on your body when you are out of control. You don't have the luxury of ignoring the problems. You can't even say you'll deal with it later. You must live and make choices and take actions in the here and now. So you try your best to stay in control and you juggle the multitude of variables.

2.3 ~ Advocates and Support

"The importance of a good friend in our life
is just like the importance of our single heartbeat!"
It's not visible, but silently supports our life."

~ Author unknown

KEY TOPICS

- Be your own very strong advocate:
  - Write down your questions and concerns,
  - Be sure you and understand the answers,
  - Ask for the best way to communicate with your healthcare provider and office staff,
  - Bring someone with you to healthcare appointments.
- It is important to have advocates for your health when in the hospital.
- Bring your advocate with you for doctor visits and trips to the hospital, when possible.
- Develop and train your team of advocates.

ADVOCATE: n. [ad-v*uh*-kit, -keyt]: *a person who speaks or writes in support or defense of a person, cause, etc.*

This is possibly the most important section of *The Savvy Diabetic: A Survival Guide.*

What do I mean? Your own health is more important and critical to you than it is to anyone else in the world. It is *survival*. There are lots of people involved in helping you be successful: doctors, CDE's, physician assistants, internet research, friends, family, support groups. But it really all boils down to you.

Communicate your concerns and needs

What could stand in your way of being your own and best advocate? Let's see.

1. "I thought the doctor was in charge."

    Well, yes, the doctor has specialized training and knowledge and certainly authority to prescribe. But it is up to you to work cooperatively with your doctor, to fully understand your own health issues, to participate in the management of your medications, and to report concerns and communicate what you need. No one could possibly know more about how you are feeling than you.

2. "I get so intimidated in the doctor's office."

    Of course, the doctor's office is his/her domain and can be very intimidating and a bit overwhelming. It is easy to get flustered and feel out of control. But try to remember that while the doctor and staff are busy running the practice, you need to get their attention and get your needs addressed.

3. "I forget to ask my questions and I don't remember what I was told."

    Yes, this happens. The best way to handle it is:

    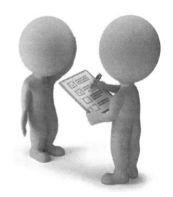

    Write down your questions before your appointment and make a copy for the doctor to work from during his/ her time with you. Consider investing in a LiveScribe SmartPen that you can use to record the visit and integrate your notes later at home on your computer.

    a. Bring your list of medications and allergies. Then, under pressure at the doctor's office, you won't have to remember what you are taking and how much.

    b. Write down important discussion issues and treatment plans. Then ask to clarify: "Let me repeat what I think I understood. is that correct?" It will reinforce what you understand and correct any misunderstandings. It is much more efficient than not being clear and then going home befuddled.

4.   "How do I get in touch with you for a question or for help?"

Every office and every healthcare provider does it differently. Ask all of your health care providers what the best way is for you to communicate with them and their office staff. Some like faxes, some prefer emails, some are set up on electronic records so that you can reach them via their portal. Be sure to ask who you go to with problems or questions. Assure them that you will only communicate with them about important issues, as you value their time.

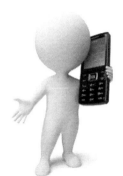

5.   "How do I get my prescriptions refilled and who do I ask?"

Prescriptions: Find out your healthcare provider's system for renewing prescriptions. Understand how they do it and make sure they know how to reach your pharmacies. This is vital. When it gets to be a hassle to renew critical medications, you can easily become frustrated and feel like giving up.

Also ask how to handle prior authorizations and denials from your insurance company. This is happening more and more frequently. You need to be able to communicate with your doctor or a designated staff person to resolve these issues.

6.   "How do I reach you with a serious concern?"

Treat your doctor's time with respect. Unless explicitly a social visit, stay focused on your concerns and needs. Keep in mind that your doctor has a busy schedule and may also encounter emergencies. If your schedule is tight, tell the office manager what your time constraints are. If your doctor often runs late, call before you arrive and ask if he/she is on time or running late. Some people prefer to be the first patient in the doctor's schedule, which reduces the chances of running behind. Ask for the best way to reach your provider, after hours, should you have an urgent or immediate need.

7. "May my spouse/friend/advocate sit in on this appointment?"

    Have an advocate. Use the team approach whenever you can. If at all possible, bring someone to serve as a second set of ears. This could be a spouse, family member, friend or someone from a support group. I have always found this to be helpful, as we can later compare notes on what we heard.

    Healthcare providers should always encourage support. If they don't, then perhaps you should ask why not, or switch to a more supportive physician.

8. "May my advocate stay with me?"

    Using a team approach is even more important if you are in the ER or hospital. There is a lot of activity in a hospital and lots of personnel coming and going and doing things with, and to, you. You are often confined to bed, so an advocate can walk to the nurses' station or get what you need more immediately.

Ask questions and get answers

It is critical to ask questions. These people are busy dealing with many patients. So ask:

➤ "What's in the IV bag?

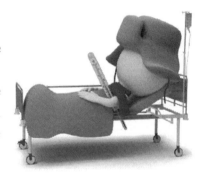

While a graduate school student, I had to go to the emergency room at the University of Pennsylvania. This was a non-diabetes-related problem and the doctor ordered an IV with electrolytes. I sat up all night, with my boyfriend at my side, waiting for the dehydration to resolve.

As we were both drowsing off, a nurse came in, at 3:00 AM to change the IV bag. We didn't think to ask about what she was administering. Around 4:00 AM, I started to feel flushed and headachy.

We called in the nurse and asked what was in the IV bag. She said, "Oh, this is just saline in a glucose solution." In a slight panic, I reached for my blood glucose meter and tested. My blood glucose was over 400!

When I asked why she gave me the glucose solution, she answered, "Well, you hadn't had any food for several hours so we often use a glucose solution." I was horrified! I said, "I am a diabetic! I can't have glucose without insulin!"

WHY IS THIS IMPORTANT AND WHAT IF I DON'T?

It may seem like a lot of prep work. But it is much easier to compile this information when you are feeling well as opposed to explaining it in the ER when you're sick, possibly in pain, and probably can't remember everything.

If you don't supply accurate information, the medical staff may give you the wrong medications, the wrong dosage, or not give you critically necessary medication.

Without proper information, mistakes can simply compound the problems you are already having.

She immediately changed out the IV bag but I learned an important lesson about IV bags and glucose or steroid mixes.

➤ "What medications are you giving me?"

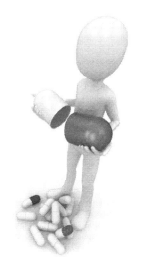

WHY IS THIS IMPORTANT AND WHAT IF I DON'T?

If you have allergies or sensitivities, make sure you explain them. Make sure the staff knows all your medications so that what they give you will not interfere or cause side effects.

➢ "I use an insulin pump. Have you seen one before?"

If you are on an insulin pump, explain your pump to the staff. I've found that they often have never seen an insulin pump and are fascinated. If you are using a continuous glucose monitor system (CGMS), that's a novelty for most. I've seen nurses call in nurses from other floors to come and see. They have even asked me to do an in service training/education. If possible, do not let them disconnect you from your pump until you have thoroughly discussed the plan to manage your blood glucose, including the type of insulin they will use.

Your support team

I can't overemphasize the importance of having an advocate, partner or support person, as your second set of ears and extra legs to get what you need. It is important for anyone being treated in the medical system. But it is essential for the diabetic, whose needs are specific, time critical, and complicated. With an advocate, in addition to yourself, you will be safer and help the medical team help you.

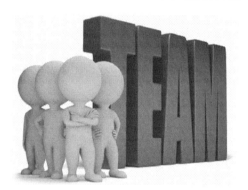

Managing diabetes on a day-to-day basis and even hour-by-hour basis means you must pay a lot of attention to your health. But if you are ill or injured, medical personnel will get involved. If you can't explain or ask, your advocate will.

Choosing an advocate

Who should you choose as an advocate? The answer is not always simple.

➢ A spouse or significant other: That's an obvious answer. Someone who lives with you, loves you, and knows your routine and your meds. Educate your partner on what you will need in case you are hospitalized.

It helps if you share your med list and dosing schedule, so your advocate can step in if you are unable, too sick, or under anesthesia. Ask your advocate to be there and actively manage the staff.

Even if you have a spouse/partner, what happens if that person is not available (i.e., out of town or in a business meeting)? Do you have a back-up support person?

➤ A family member or friend: Same applies here. Share with them your med list, dosing schedule and your needs/concerns for managing your daily health. Ask if this person can step in if you need help. Be prepared to help him or her understand what your medical conditions are and what you need done for you. But also be prepared to deal with his or her hesitation and help your advocate understand how valuable he or she is to you.

This can be a very uncomfortable concept. It is very difficult for me, too. I generally manage my health and don't talk to a lot of friends about what I do on a daily basis. I always worry that if I ask for help, my friends will back away or be frightened, as if the task is too large. I have one close friend who is also a physician so he doesn't need too much prep. However, I also have a close girlfriend who has access to my medical lists and knows who to contact for additional support.

This may be too difficult for some friends. Be prepared for someone to be reticent or actually decline. It's better to know this before you need help and expect that friend to step in. Assess this carefully, as this person could be your lifeline. You need to know he/she is on board and there for you.

As I write this, I realize how difficult this step is. It causes me a lot of discomfort and I just want to ignore it. But the reality is that the better prepared you are with support, the safer you will be in a medical setting.

➤ A member of a support group: This is similar to asking a friend. But he/she might have special knowledge of diabetes management and be available if you need help with either a doctor's appointment or trip to the hospital.

Train your advocate to be successful

Make sure your advocate wants to help. This is really an important point. You may have many good friends but you are looking for friends who are willing to take the time to understand your needs and step up when you are not able to speak for yourself. Not all your friends or family will feel comfortable or have the skill set to be your voice in the stress of a doctor's office or in the hubbub of the hospital.

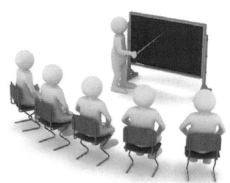

> ➤ Share your medical concerns and information so he or she knows enough about you, your conditions, and your medications to be of help to you.[SB coach]

> ➤ Encourage your advocate to be gently persistent. The more that advocate is liked and listened to, the more effective your care will be. Any doctor's office or hospital can be frustrating. But remind your advocate that the staff is managing many divergent tasks and claims on their time. Remind your advocate to be as pleasant and direct as possible, find out what he or she can do without needing to interrupt the staff (find out where the blankets are, how to get water, etc.), and be sure to be nice and show appreciation for his or her help.

> ➤ As you explain and encourage your advocate, be aware, and help him or her to be aware of how much time and effort it takes for you to be a diabetic. In the next chapter, we'll discuss the time commitment you make, each and every day, controlling, juggling, and managing what most people (non-diabetics) take for granted.

> ➤ Advocate practice and training time is essential. You will need to show your advocate(s) how you manage your diabetes and exactly what you will need them to do to help you. See the appendix for some thoughts on training your advocate to help you. But here are some critical questions to address.

>> ✧ Does your advocate know how to:

>> ✧ Listen carefully and ask intelligent questions?

>> ✧ Fill a syringe with insulin?

- ✧ Manage your insulin pump?
- ✧ Operate your CGMS?
- ✧ Test your blood glucose?
- ✧ Find and read your medication list?
- ✧ Contact your emergency contacts ?
- ✧ Contact your doctors?

➢ Show GREAT appreciation for your advocate. It truly does take a lot of time, thought, and action to manage your health. When he or she helps you, show that you are aware of how much effort is involved.

"I had been told that the training procedure with cats was difficult.
It's not. Mine had me trained in two days."

~ Bill Dana, American comedian, actor and screenwriter

A QUICK REVIEW OF KEY TOPICS:
ADVOCATES AND SUPPORT

- Be your own very strong advocate:
  - Write down your questions and concerns, and be sure you and understand the answers.
  - Ask for the best way to communicate with your healthcare provider and office staff regarding:
    - Health issues and illnesses,
    - Prescription refills and requests,
    - Medical questions.
  - Bring someone with you to healthcare appointments.
- Bring your advocate with you for doctor visits and trips to the hospital, if possible, using a team approach.
- It is critically important to have advocates to be your voice and extra set of ears when in the hospital.
  - Develop and train your team of advocates. Determine who is willing and available, if you need help.
  - Explain how you manage your health and what you will need them to do for you.
  - Educate them and support them.

PART 3: DAY TO DAY, 24/7

3.1 Choosing your Medical Team

    ✧ How to choose your doctor

    ✧ Checklist of doctor and medical practice characteristics

    ✧ Interviewing your doctors

    ✧ Questions to ask potential endocrinologists

    ✧ Resources to learn more about doctors in your area

3.2 Hypoglycemia, Hyperglycemia and Unawareness

3.3 Time: How much time does it take to have diabetes?

3.4 Your Medical Information

    ✧ Your Basic Information

    ✧ Your Medications and Allergies

    ✧ List of Emergency Contacts and Medical Team

3.5 Visits: the Doctor, the Lab and Radiology

3.6 Natural Disasters: Earthquakes, Tornadoes, Hurricanes and Floods

3.1 ~ Choosing Your Medical Team

"Whenever a doctor cannot do good,
he must be kept from doing harm."

~ *Hippocrates, ancient Greek physician*

KEY TOPICS:

- Identify your own criteria for choosing a doctor.
- Evaluate the doctor's office to meet your needs (including ease of communications, auxiliary staff availability, location).
- Interview questions to ask a potential doctor.
- Resources to help you find your dream medical team.

TEAM, n. [teem]: a number of persons associated in some joint action: a team of advisers.

I had the routine pediatric doctors and other childhood specialties. But at age 11, my world changed. Over the 48 years I've had Type 1 diabetes, I have lived in seven different states, and I'd estimate that I've been treated by well over 100 doctors of various specialties across those different locations.

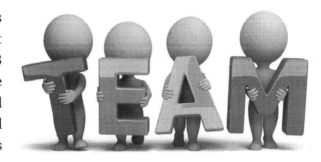

At age 11, I needed an endocrinologist, and relied on my parents to choose the doctor based on his philosophy of diabetes management and how they could interact with him. At that time, much less was known about complications and control.

I became a patient of one of the top endocrinologists, Dr. Henry Dolger, who practiced in New York City (a half hour drive for us) and had written one of the well-regarded books on managing diabetes, called How to Live with Diabetes, published in 1958 (seven years before I was diagnosed). He was considered the guru for diabetics. His assistant would come to get me in the waiting room and say loudly, "Come, let me stick you." It caused me so much anxiety, every time. My young, 11-year-old mind heard that this lady wanted to hurt me and she sounded gleeful about it. To this day, I can still hear her shrill voice and feel my instinct to run away.

When the nurse was done sticking my finger, the doctor would breeze in, talking about his diabetic patients all over the world who were doing all sorts of wild and wondrous adventures. I'm sure he was trying to make me feel hopeful. It made Mom feel optimistic but I did not feel encouraged. Then he promised me that there would be a cure for diabetes in two years. So, two years later, in 1967, he promised me a cure in five years. He had lied to me, and I lost faith: in him, in doctors, and in the hope for a cure.

The worst part of my experience with Dr. Dolger was his approach to diabetes management. He mostly feared low blood glucose, so all of us patients were taught that it was just fine to have high blood glucose. A whole generation of diabetics under his care didn't worry about control.

Dr. Dolger was not alone is this thinking. Indeed, this was the general thinking of the majority of physicians and medical practices at that time (in the 1950-1970 timeframe). Dr. Dolger changed his teachings in the mid-1980s but that was long after so many suffered complications. I personally lost three good friends to complications of diabetes before they reached the joyful age of 30. It was so wrong and so sad.

"It is a mathematical fact that fifty percent of all doctors
graduate in the bottom half of their class."
~ Author unknown

How to choose your doctors

Usually a key member of your medical team will be an endocrinologist, although often a knowledgeable internist can help with diabetes management. What do you look for? What is important to you and what are your options?

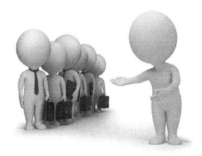

TIP **Choose a Team Leader**	This is the time to be aware of and perhaps determine how your team works. Usually, a team has a team leader. Usually the leader is the primary care physician or internal medical doctor.

However, since diabetes is such an integral part of your medical condition, very often, the team leader might be your endocrinologist. On the other hand, your endocrinologist may only want to treat you for your diabetes issues and defer the common cold to a generalist.

How do you know and what do you prefer? If you want your endocrinologist to be in charge, let him or her know that and find out if he or she is willing to serve as both diabetes specialist and primary care provider. If not, he or she may recommend an internist (specialist in internal medicine) to head up the team and be the go-to person for routine issues.

It helps to understand what you are looking for in a doctor. Below is a list of characteristics and features someone might want in his or her physician. Remember, not everyone has the same criteria but it is helpful to know what is important to you.

"If I could solve all the problems myself, I would."
~ *Thomas Edison, American inventor and businessman*

Checklist of Doctor and Medical Practice Characteristics

Office and Location
- Distance from home or office
- Ease of parking
- Ambiance of waiting room
- Ambiance and cleanliness of facilities

Doctor Qualifications
- Education, board specialty and certification
- Years in practice
- Reputation
- Research-based
- Hospital affiliation
- Has good referrals from patients and from doctors
- Offers good referrals out to other specialists

Office & Practice
- Keeps appointments usually within 15 minutes
- Gives you as much time as you need
- Friendly and quick check-in and check-out
- Takes your medical insurance
- Fast response on refills
- Phone calls / emails returned promptly
- Who handles office visits: Doctor? Physician assistant? Nurse practitioner?
- Partners and coverage after hours and on weekends
- After hours contact for emergencies
- Provides copies of labs to patient
- Online records and labs
- Online prescription renewal

Personal Characteristics
- Certain and knowledgeable
- Up-to-date on latest information and technologies
- Warm and compassionate demeanor
- Socially engaging
- Empathetic to your circumstances
- Interested in holistic life and family

"I recently went to a new doctor and noticed he was located in something called the Professional Building. I felt better right away."

~ George Carlin, American stand-up comedian, social critic, satirist, actor, writer/author

As you look through this list, you can circle those items that seem most important to you. Rate them in order of importance (1–10) and pay attention to the items with the highest ratings as you review your choices of physician.

You should also assess the doctor's office staff for qualities important for you, as they will be the people you will have to interact with.

Interviewing your doctor

You can, and should, ask to meet the endocrinologist (or any doctor) before you choose to become a patient. Most often, they will give you 15 minutes to meet and see if you will fit in well with him/her and the practice.

What do you say? What do you want to know? What do you ask?

Here are some questions you might want to ask when choosing a doctor as a part of your medical team. Remember, when you ask questions, the doctor sees that you will be an active participant in your own care, which makes both you and the doctor successful.

Questions to Ask Potential Endocrinologists / Healthcare Providers *

- What is your experience with Type 1 or Type 2 Diabetes?
- Where would you expect my HbA1c's to average?
- How often do you see Type 1 or Type 2 Diabetics?
- How long are your visits?
- Do often do you request HbA1c? Do you test HbA1c in your office?
- How many times a day do you expect me to test my blood sugar?
- What is your protocol on treating a low blood sugar?

- What is your protocol on treating a blood sugar >300?
- When do you have your patient's test ketones?
- When would you recommend Glucagon?
- Do you have a CDE who is experienced with Type 1? Type 2? Type 1.5?
- Do you have a dietician who is experienced in Type 1? Type2? Type 1.5?
- Who takes insulin adjustment calls and what are the hours?
- Who do I call in the middle of the night?
- What do I do if I get sick?
- Are you familiar with all the insulin pumps on the market?
- Do you know how to adjust pumps?
- Do you download pumps and meters at every visit?
- Do you have many patients on CGMS?
- Who does your prior authorizations should I have an issue with supplies?

~ Thanks to Elizabeth Beko, BSN, RN, CDE, CHOC Children's Specialty Center at the Mary and Dick Allen Diabetes Center, Newport Beach, CA, for sharing this list with me.

Other resources to help you find a great doctor

> **Support Groups**: Members of a diabetes support group can give you great information. Always consider asking other diabetics, "Who's your endocrinologist? Are you satisfied/happy? Why or why not?"

> **Sales Reps**: Another excellent resource for feedback on doctors and medical practices are sales representatives for diabetes products and supplies. If you talk with the sales representatives, ask them which doctors they think are the best and why. They tend to know the doctors and offices well and will probably give you some very insightful feedback.

Your options for doctors may be limited by where you live. If you are in a rural area, there may only be one endocrinologist nearby or maybe none. If that's the case, you will have to make the best of the situation and develop a good relationship with that physician.

However, if you do have choices, the checklist of doctor and practice characteristics, as well as the list of questions for an interview, will help you focus on the best medical team member for your needs.

Use this evaluation system and these questions for the rest of the medical team (cardiologist, certified diabetes educator, neurologist, nephrologist, ophthalmologist, gastroenterologist, podiatrist, gynecologist, urologist, and any others you may need).

Tell them where they are on the team and who to copy on their results. Tell your lead doctor who all your support doctors are.

Since we have to deal with doctors, it is important that we like and feel comfortable with our team as best as possible and understand how to work effectively with them.

A QUICK REVIEW OF KEY TOPICS:
CHOOSING YOUR MEDICAL TEAM

- Decide what criteria you need in choosing and working with a doctor or healthcare provider.
- Evaluate the healthcare provider and the medical office environment and staff, based on our needs, including:
  - Access to office, doctor and staff,
  - "Personality" of the office.
- Review the Interview Questions to ask a potential medical team.
- Use all the resources available to you to find the best medical team:
  - Diabetes and insulin pump support groups,
  - Diabetes sales representatives and sales support staff:
    - Ask for their referrals and cautions,
    - Ask for their assessment of the healthcare provider's knowledge, personality, accessibility.

3.2 ~ Hypoglycemia, Hyperglycemia and Unawareness

"Sugar in the gourd and honey in the horn,
I was so happy since the hour I was born."
~ Author unknown

KEY TOPICS

- Discuss with your doctor about his/her guidelines for diabetes control.
- Consider using a continuous glucose monitoring system (CGMS).
- Try to avoid too many low blood glucose episodes.

HYPOGLYCEMIA: n. [hi-poh-glahy-see-mee-uh]: *an abnormally low level of glucose in the blood.*

HYPERGLYCEMIA: n.[hi-per-glahy-see-mee-*uh*]: *an abnormally high level of glucose in the blood.*

UNAWARENESS: n. [uhn-*uh*-wair nis]: *not aware or conscious; unconscious*

The causes and mechanisms of diabetes are complex, and so much is unknown. Indeed, a researcher at the University of California, Irvine, recently stated that the pancreas is an angry organ and it is the second most complicated part of the body after the brain.

But here's what we do know:

In Type 1 diabetes, the body does not produce insulin, which regulates or metabolizes glucose in the cells. Therefore, we take insulin, trying to mimic what a healthy body does automatically. Our ability to maintain balance has so many variables and changes from day to day. But we do our best, using insulin, measuring carbs, incorporating exercise, and managing stress (both from illness and emotions).

In Type 2 diabetes, the most common form of diabetes, either the body does not produce enough insulin or the cells ignore the insulin. Insulin is necessary for the body to be able to convert glucose to energy.

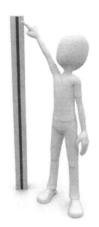

The measure of our success is our blood glucose levels. We don't want too many lows or too many highs or too much variability (up and down). It is essentially our job as diabetics to minimize hypoglycemia and hyperglycemia. This by far makes up the longest segment of time in managing diabetes. Many diabetics are committed to keeping diabetes under control. Surviving with diabetes is a skill set which allows us to overcome challenges and plan our time effectively.

What happens when our blood glucose goes too low?

- Shaky
- Sweaty
- Confused
- Argumentative
- Edgy
- Dizzy
- Hungry
- Pale
- Racing heart
- Poor coordination and more

Left untreated, low blood glucose can lead to convulsions, coma and death.

That certainly gets your attention, doesn't it?

What happens when our blood glucose goes too high?

➤ Thirst

➤ Drowsiness and lethargy

➤ Vision changes

➤ Labored breathing

➤ Frequent urination

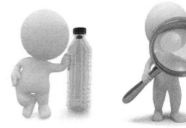

And left untreated, high blood glucose can lead to stupor, coma, and death.

Again, got your attention? This is the balancing act for a diabetic.

But wait, there's more! As Type 1 diabetics live longer (and especially for females), studies have shown that they run an increased chance to develop hypoglycemia and hyperglycemia unawareness (in which they do not get the normal warning signs of low or high blood glucose).

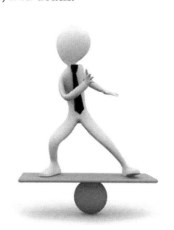

Does this sound frightening?

It is. That risk comes with the warning of sudden death, or what so unkindly is referred to as dead in bed syndrome. This can occur when our blood glucose drops precipitously during the night, and without warning cues, we can sleep on through into coma and death.

This is scary!

What can we do? According to Dr. Steve Edelman (endocrinologist in San Diego, founder of Taking Control of Your Diabetes, and a Type 1 diabetic himself), there are four predisposing conditions that you can do something about.

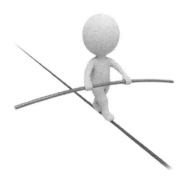

➤ Ease up on the tight blood glucose control. If your HbA1c tends to run at or below 6, you may be experiencing too many low blood glucose episodes.

You might be better to relax your control to about 6.5–7.0. Discuss this with your doctor as it could save your life.

➢ Avoid nighttime low blood glucose. This is a tricky problem, but the best advice is to use a CGMS which can alert you if your blood glucose drops suddenly or seriously low. It is a difficult tightrope to walk. Don't go too low, don't go too high, and don't wobble too much.

➢ If you do not wake from the CGMS receiver alerts, place the receiver in a glass on your nightstand. The noise of it vibrating in the glass will probably get you up.

➢ You are best not to sleep alone. What does this mean? You are safer if you have a spouse, significant other, or roommate. Is this a reason to be in a relationship? No, but it underscores the absolute critical need for an advocate, someone in your life who can step in and help you when you are less than able to complete these life essential daily tasks.

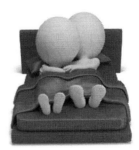

"I have a new philosophy.
I'm only going to dread one day at a time."
~ *Charles Schultz, American cartoonist*

A QUICK REVIEW OF KEY TOPICS:
HYPOGLYCEMIA, HYPERGLYCEMIA AND UNAWARENESS

- Discuss with your doctor how tight your control should be, ideally.
- Consider using a continuous glucose monitoring system to alert you of:
  - Low blood glucose episodes,
  - High blood glucose episodes,
  - Rapidly dropping or rising glucose.
- Try to avoid too many low blood glucose episodes.

3.3 ~ Time: How much time does it take to have diabetes?

"The only reason for time is so that everything doesn't happen at once."
~ *Albert Einstein, German born American physicist*

KEY TOPIC

- Living with diabetes consumes a lot of time, really!

How much time does it take to manage diabetes? This is a very interesting exercise!

To be a good diabetic, I have to:

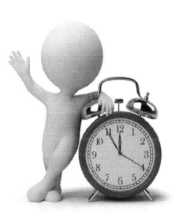

- ➤ Monitor my blood glucose,
- ➤ Take insulin,
- ➤ Figure out how many carbs are in my food,
- ➤ Calculate the proper amount of insulin to cover my carb,
- ➤ Be aware of high blood glucose and low blood glucose,
- ➤ Order, and maintain, prescriptions,
- ➤ Treat low blood glucose episodes,
- ➤ Change infusion sets and reservoir,
- ➤ Change CGMS sensor,
- ➤ Go to doctors and other healthcare providers,
- ➤ Go to labs,
- ➤ Go to pharmacies, [Managing diabetes]
- ➤ Following up on insurance claims,
- ➤ Analyze glucose readings.

So how much time does it take to manage diabetes? Without feeling sorry for ourselves, let's just take a look. Bear in mind, as you read this that this is why it is so important to have a strong support system.

Testing

The average meter takes five seconds once the blood hits the strip to give you a reading. Adding in the time for finding the meter, loading it, reading the result, and cleaning up afterwards, it takes about one minute each time you test. Do that eight times a day (at least) and you now have used up eight minutes a day. Do that every day for a year and blood testing takes more than 48 hours a year.

Changing needles or changing infusion sets, and taking insulin

Changing a needle on an insulin pen takes, on average, six seconds per needle. Add in the time it takes to remove/dispose of the needle, uncap/attach the new needle, and fill the syringe or dial in the pen dosage, and you are looking at two minutes. If you are injecting five times a day (and actually changing the needle), that means 10 minutes a day. Over the course of a year, that amounts to over 60 hours of giving the life-saving medication that keeps going

Changing insulin pump infusion sets can take even more time than shots, but you only do that every few days. None the less, you may be adjusting your pump settings up to 10 times a day to account for meal bolus or adjustments for exercise, of high/ low blood glucose readings. So let's just stick with the same 60 hours a year to administer insulin.

Going to your doctor/healthcare provider

Typically, the average diabetic (who is well controlled) will see their endocrinologist once every three to six months and it may include a visit to the certified diabetes educator (CDE), as well. After wait times, the actual consult (typically 30 minutes, in my experience) including driving and parking, takes around two hours per visit. So with four visits per year, we spend eight hours getting the information we need, only half of which is spent actually seeing the doctor. Assuming we see at least two more doctors related to diabetes, let's add another 8 hours with healthcare folks for a total of 16 hours per year.

Getting lab work done

This is probably the least fun of all the things we do. Getting a needle in the vein never feels good and, for the privilege, we spend at least 40 minutes (wait time included), four times a year to find out our and other significant lab values. Add to that another 20 minutes to get the results from the lab or doctor's office and you've spent 4 hours each year to confirm you are on the right track.

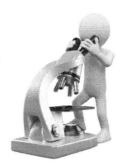

Going to the pharmacy to get your supplies

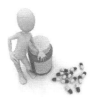

Once every two months, I need to get something diabetes-related from the pharmacy. Spending an average of 30 minutes each time (including drive time, ordering online, or requesting refills from the doctor's office) amounts to 6 hours per year getting necessary supplies.

Treating hypoglycemia (low blood glucose)

If ever there is a time that diabetes gives some enjoyment, this could be it; I don't mean the actual hypoglycemia, I mean eating sweet things to raise the blood glucose. Hypoglycemia costs us 25 minutes (factoring in waiting for the blood glucose to rise, testing, and actually eating the sugar). A well-controlled diabetic (according to endocrinologists) is having 0-1 mild low blood glucose episodes a week. Rounding it up to two per week, that gives us over 1 hour a week treating hypoglycemia, and over a year, it comes to over 52 hours managing low blood glucose. Naturally, we want to avoid these as much as possible, and if there was ever a place to save time, this is by far the biggest.

Treating hyperglycemia (high blood glucose)

Now, this is an interesting one. Let's say we define this as a blood glucose reading over 250. First there is the calculation to add extra insulin, administer it, and wait for your blood glucose to come down, including all the retesting. For each hyperglycemia episode, allow two hours. If this happens once a week, managing it comes to almost 104 hours per year managing hyperglycemic episodes and feeling not so great.

Following up on insurance claims and filling out forms

These are probably the most frustrating and time-consuming of all things concerning diabetes. This includes getting prior authorizations, refills, and out-of-network issues, it takes around 30 minutes including printing forms and sending them in. Do this once every month and add in two phone calls at 30 minutes (including hold time). You have spent 18 hours of your life that you will never get back.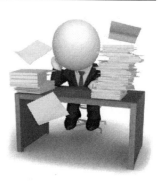

Analyzing results

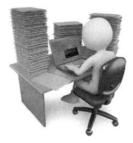 At least once a month, I take a look at my glucose records to see how I'm doing. Feedback (good or bad) is how we improve, and the body is continually changing its requirements. It is not until we analyze how we are doing that we can optimize our own care. With that in mind, it's safe to say we spend one hour per month or 12 hours a year of ensuring optimal care.

Food, eating, and insulin

Calculating the amount of insulin a particular meal deserves some careful review. This is a deceptively significant amount of time, including:

- ➢ Deciding what you plan to eat,
- ➢ Figuring out how many carbs are in the food,
- ➢ Evaluating the glycemic index of that food,
- ➢ Calculating the fat content, which impacts how quickly or slowly you will need the insulin delivered,
- ➢ Recalculating, after the meal, if you misjudged the carbs,

➤ If you are eating out or on an airplane, trying to guess when the food will be delivered, whether you will like it and eat all or a portion of it, and trying to assess the amounts of hidden sugars in the food,

➤ Adjusting your dosage for deciding to eat that extra piece of bread or sample the dessert,

➤ Accounting for any intake of wine, beer or other alcoholic drinks,

➤ The time you spend making diabetes-related decisions, such as the need to take additional insulin and the constant evaluation of "how am I feeling?"

Let's take a guess at this. I'm guessing we spend three minutes per meal plus snacks. That amounts to 12 minutes per day spent figuring and calculating food consumption and insulin requirements usually all in our heads. That adds up to 79 hours per year, just doing the math.

Miscellaneous other stuff

And there is MORE!

Let's not forget about the time it takes to:

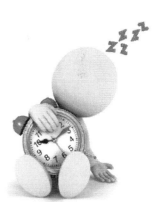

➤ Call tech support about your pump or CGMS (which always takes longer than you planned),

➤ File appeals (which means talking to your doctor's office, pharmacy, and insurance companies),

➤ Change CGM sensors,

➤ Be concerned about little things like a cut on your toe that you'd hardly notice if you didn't have diabetes,

➤ Think about whether to pull an infusion set vs. giving it a little longer to see if that last correction is going to kick in soon,

➤ Explain stuff to or educating the diabetes police, the food police, the curious, or even just someone who cares,

➤ See extra visits to eye doctors, podiatrists and the whole line-up of specialists that you would never have met if you had a perfectly functioning pancreas.

So, let's give this all a number—conservatively, 10 minutes a day or 61 hours a year of your life handling the extra stuff that comes with having diabetes!

"It does not do to leave a live dragon out of your calculations,
if you live near him."

~ *JRR Tolkien, English writer (The Hobbit), poet, philologist and professor*

All added up, how much time do we spend taking care of our diabetes?

Let's do the math.

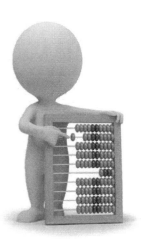

Testing blood glucose	48 hr/yr
Changing needles, infusion sets, taking shots	60 hr/yr
Doctor Appointments	16 hr/yr
Going to the Laboratory	4 hr/yr
Dealing with the Pharmacy and RX renewals	6 hr/yr
Managing Hypoglycemia	52 hr/yr
Correcting Hyperglycemia	104 hr/yr
Dealing with Insurance Issues	18 hr/yr
Analysis/Correction of blood glucose data	12 hr/yr
Calculating Food and Insulin	79 hr/yr
Miscellaneous	61 hr/yr

**Total: 460 hours/year, or
8.9 hours/week, or
57.5 work days per year**

Just to help you put this in perspective: If you spend 10 minutes each day blow-drying your hair or shaving, that's 1.2 hours a week in just daily grooming. Just imagine your life if you had to spend 80 minutes per day (spread out throughout the day) blow drying your hair or shaving.

My thanks in this section to: Harrison Hughes of The Diabetic Skill Set focusing on T1 skills, curediabetesblog.com and DebM555, moderator of the DiabetesCGMS Yahoo User Forum, as well as a T1

Perhaps, upon being diagnosed with diabetes, one should borrow the creed from the United States Postal Service:

"Neither snow nor rain nor heat nor gloom of night
stays these couriers from the swift completion
of their appointed rounds."
~ *Inscription on the James Farley Post Office in New York City*

How do I feel about having diabetes? Without applying for, or wanting it, I was assigned a 24/7 job that I never get paid for. In fact, I have to pay to keep it. And I can never quit or call in sick or take a vacation from it, either.

Others usually do not understand or appreciate my job (although they often think they do and therefore feel free to share their misunderstandings and uninformed opinions about it). And I am continuously being told that "there will be a cure any day now" and then this job will no longer exist. I have been hearing this for 16 years.

Casey O., Type 1 diabetes for 16 years

❧

"Put your hand on a hot stove for a minute, and it seems like an hour. Sit with a pretty girl for an hour, and it seems like a minute. THAT'S relativity."

~ Albert Einstein, German-born American theoretical physicist

❧

A QUICK REVIEW OF KEY TOPICS: TIME

- If you feel like living with diabetes consumes a lot of your time, you are RIGHT! Could be 9 hours/week, more or less!
- Try your own exercise of adding up the time it takes to be you with diabetes.

3.4 ~ Your Medical Information

"The original lists were probably carved in stone and represented
longer periods of time. They contained things like
'Get More Clay. Make Better Oven' "

~ David Viscott, American psychologist and radio personality

KEY TOPICS

- Be prepared not for if but for when the unexpected happens
- Make lists and update often. Include your medical information, schedule of medications and your emergency and medical contacts

---

I always worried that I could end up in the hospital or the ER, and at the mercy of medical personnel who may not know how to manage my diabetes, or simply just be too busy.

As I mentioned at the beginning of the book, my bout with appendicitis was totally unplanned (of course), and I certainly couldn't have predicted my trip to the hospital nor chosen a much worse scenario:

> - out of town,
> - on a holiday weekend,
> - under time pressure,
> - busy,
> - in pain.

I had a few good things on my side:

> - I was in the US (people spoke English),
> - my husband was with me,
> - he knew my medical conditions and medications.

While waiting for my doctor to call me, we made a list on my husband's laptop of all the medications I could remember, and all my doctor contacts, all the while gripping my increasingly painful abdomen. We then linked into the hotel network and printed my lists via the business office.

We arrived at the emergency room around 10:00 PM on one of the busiest nights in their history. Since I was not bleeding or violently ill (at least not yet), we were told to wait: so we waited and waited. Around 4:00 AM, I was in-processed, placed on a gurney and parked in a hallway, since all the rooms were full. I had forgotten to bring snacks so we only had vending machine candy for food to sustain us.

It was then that I realized that I just wasn't prepared.

～

"When the student is ready, the master appears."
~ Buddhist Proverb

～

PREPARED: adj. [priˈpe(ə)r/d]:

    1. Made (something) ready for use or consideration

    2. Created in advance; preplanned

OK, I survived that stay. Within 18 hours of my first pains, my appendix left my body, and within 22 hours of my surgery, I left the hospital. Amazing! []

But I still had more lessons to learn.

Again, on another dark and stormy night two years later, I needed to go to the ER near my home with a kidney infection and developing pneumonia — again not diabetes related, but urgent. Fortunately, I was at home at the time and could print my medications list. I was admitted to the hospital directly from the ER, but I still wasn't prepared for a six-day stay in the hospital. I didn't know what to bring or how to manage my food. I felt very off-balance and out of control.

It occurred to me that perhaps I could get wiser and more prepared, if it ever happened again. *Then I convinced myself that it wouldn't happen again. Silly me!*

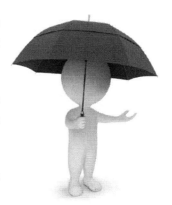

It happened again! Within a year, another trip to the ER with three days in the hospital on, and would you believe it, it was another dark and stormy night!

Then another time, I needed major surgery, with four days in the intensive care unit.

It was beginning to dawn on me that I needed to do this better. With my growing experience with hospital settings, perhaps I could share what I had learned painfully through my mistakes.

"Now my troubles are going to have troubles with me!
I have heard there are troubles of more than one kind.
Some come from ahead and some come from behind.
But I've bought a big bat. I'm all ready, you see.
Now my troubles are going to have troubles with me!"
~ *Dr. Seuss, American writer, poet and cartoonist*

So here we go!

Remember, in The Essentials: Basic Steps to Survival, we talked about making lists? I cannot emphasize enough the critical importance of having your information listed.

What should my lists look like? I've included what I use, as an example, along with another possible format, in Part Eight: Appendix. Feel free to make it yours. If possible, include a copy of your most recent lab results, which you can keep in a scanned pdf format as well as hard copy.

And what do you do with these lists? As we talked about earlier, bring a printed copy with you when going to the hospital, emergency room, urgent care, or when you are away from home (business or vacation). You can keep a copy of the file on a flash drive, attached to your keychain/house keys. If you are a technology person, you can also store this information, password protected, in the cloud.

"Learn from the mistakes of others.
You can never live long enough to make them all yourself."
~ John Luther, American lawyer and writer

A QUICK REVIEW OF KEY TOPICS:
YOUR MEDICAL INFORMATION

- Be prepared just in case the unexpected happens, when you least expect it!
- Make lists
  - Your medical information, including:
    - Health conditions,
    - Allergies,
    - Medications, dosages and schedule when you take them.
  - Be sure to identify medications and supplements that are critical or essential.
  - Keep a detailed list of emergency contacts, your medical teams, your identification card and your insurance cards.

3.5 ~ Visits to the Doctor, the Lab and Radiology

"Some people think that doctors and nurses can put
scrambled eggs back in the shell."

~ Cass Canfield, American publishing executive

KEY TOPICS

- Bring current medication list and most recent lab results along with questions and concerns (and pen and paper to write answers).
- Call ahead to see if your doctor is on time or running late.
- Remember that your doctors are busy and working as best as possible to see their patients.
- Use your best skills for staying calm and patient.

CONTROL ~ we keep coming back to the issue of maintaining control. This remains true when dealing with your doctors, the laboratory, and radiology.

Remember our basic steps:

➤ Be proactive,

➤ Be prepared,

➤ Ask questions,

➤ Communicate,

➤ Be your own best advocate,

➤ Bring an advocate with you.

You have diabetes. You know what you do to take care of yourself. But when you are in a medical setting, it can feel like you have lost your power. Here are some steps to help empower you.

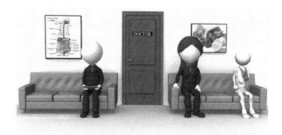

Appointment with Your Doctor

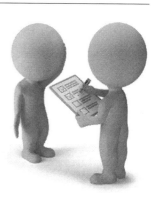

- ➤ Make your medical list. This means:
    - ✧ List of all your medications and supplements,
    - ✧ Indicate dosages (how much and when you take each),
    - ✧ List all your surgeries and any issues,
- ➤ Detail any allergies and reactions.
- ➤ Bring a copy of your latest lab work, if you have it.
- ➤ Make two copies of your written list of questions and concerns. Give one to your doctor and keep one for yourself, along with a pen to make notes.
- ➤ If you expect you might have some issues or weighty concerns, it is always helpful to have a second set of ears. If possible, bring someone you trust to listen and ask appropriate and useful questions.
- ➤ It is frequently helpful to be able to contact your doctor, to clarify any issues and concerns that may pop into your head after your visit. Be sure you know how to contact your doctor or staff (electronic medical records portal, email, fax, voicemail, medical assistant). Reassure your doctor that you will only use this contact for important issues, not to chit chat or send jokes.

❧

"Never go to a doctor whose office plants have died."
~ *Erma Bombeck, American humorist*

❧

Trip to the lab

Going to the laboratory is a fact of life for diabetics. Usually our lab tests will need to be done fasting (i.e., before you get any food or coffee). Here are some tips to expedite the process.

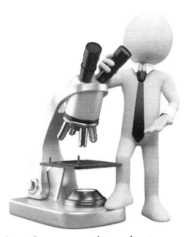

➤ Be sure to bring your insurance card, driver's license and lab slip. If possible, make a copy of the lab slip for your files, in case there are errors by the lab.

➤ If you are fasting, no coffee or juice, breakfast or snack. Ask your medical team if you should also wait before taking medications, such as thyroid or other meds.

➤ If you are on an insulin pump, you can let your regular basal rate continue, just skip the breakfast bolus (boost of insulin for a meal) or shot of insulin, until your lab work is done. Check with your doctor or certified diabetes educator for their instructions.

    ✧ If you take insulin injections, check with your doctor about whether you should:

        ✛ take your long-acting morning insulin, but certainly no insulin for breakfast, or

        ✛ wait to take all your insulin until you plan to eat.

➤ Labs can be very busy first thing in the morning. That translates into long wait times. I've also found the lab waiting room to be a little emptier very early on Monday mornings. It's after the weekend and many patients haven't seen their doctors yet for the week. This is not a hard and fast rule, but worth asking your lab techs.

- ➤ Some labs let you make appointments. If possible, choose that option. Usually the lab will take you within 10 minutes of your appointment time.

- ➤ If you go to the same lab for all your lab needs, make friends with the staff. They will take the best care of you and even get you copies of your results, after your doctor has reviewed and approved them for release. You can ask what days/times are less busy for them.

- ➤ Check your blood glucose, if necessary, or watch your CGMS. If you see your blood glucose dropping, you can take a sugar cube or let the lab staff know you are having blood glucose problem.

- ➤ While your time in the waiting room can seem wildly frustrating, remember that most labs are run as a first come, first serve system. It doesn't help to get angry at the lab technicians. They can't take you before someone ahead of you.

So it is best to just be prepared, watch your blood glucose, try to go at less busy times, and practice being meditative, read a good book, or listen to music.

Visit to Radiology: X-rays, CT scans and MRIs

Radiology departments and imaging centers also often work on a first come, first serve basis for x-rays. Give them a call ahead of your visit and ask for the wait time. At least you can be prepared and bring a snack in case you might need one.

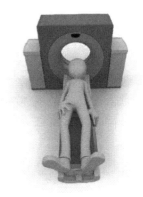

CT scans and MRI's can often be done by appointment. That is helpful but I've found that they often run later than the appointed time. Again, bring a snack and something to read, to help pass the time.

CT scans are often done with contrast. You should always let the techs know that you are a diabetic. If you have to drink a contrast (dye) drink, verify that there is no sugar added.

MRI's and insulin pumps and CGMS don't go well together. Usually the intake reps will ask about infusion pumps or other metals in your body.

- ➢ If you use a pump with tubing, you can usually leave the infusion set in your site but remove the pump and leave it in the dressing area.

- ➢ If you are using a pod pump, you will have to remove the pod and start a new one when you have finished your MRI. Check with your pod company as they may replace the pod that you have to remove.

- ➢ If you are connected to a CGMS, you will also have to remove that and put in a new sensor after the MRI.

Always ask how long the tests should take. If it is longer than a ½ hour, you might want to bolus a little before you disconnect your pump and test your blood glucose immediately after your MRI, as your blood glucose might be rising.

It sure does take a bit more work to be a diabetic in a lab or radiology setting. But with a little planning, it becomes much more manageable.

I have designed a workbook that should help keep you, your medical records and your information organized. Called *The Savvy Diabetic: On The Go*, it comes in 2 versions. One is a complete hardcopy workbook for you to use immediately to keep all your important information, latest labs, test, etc., and a prep sheet for upcoming appointments. The other is a download file for you to put together your own workbook, with instructions on how to organize your *The Savvy Diabetic: On The Go* book, how to buy the inserts you need and downloadable and editable forms to keep your workbook up to date. *The Savvy Diabetic: On The Go* is available on www.TheSavvyDiabetic.com!

∽

"When I told my doctor I couldn't afford an operation,
he offered to touch-up my X-rays."
~ *Henny Youngman, American comedian*

∽

A Quick Review of Key Topics:
Visits Doctor, Lab and Radiology

- For your visit to your healthcare provider, bring:
  - Your updated of current medication,
  - Notes of questions and concerns and follow up issues,
  - Pen and paper,
  - Most recent lab results.
- If you are on a tight time schedule, call ahead to find out the wait times to see the doctor or to complete your labs and x-rays.
- Try to remember that all your health professionals are usually working as efficiently as they can and that there may be delays.
- Bring a book, music or just your best skills for staying calm and patient.

3.6 ~ Natural Disasters: Earthquakes, Tornadoes, Hurricanes and Floods

"Weather forecast for tonight: dark.
Continued dark overnight,
with widely scattered light by morning."
~ George Carlin, American comedian and actor

KEY TOPICS

- **Be Prepared!**
- If you live in an area subject to natural disasters, keep extra insulin and other critical medications and supplies nearby, plus snacks, water, and a hard copy of your medical lists.

Natural disasters are just that. Natural, unexpected and potentially disastrous.

If you live in an area where these acts of God can happen, it is even more important for you to be prepared. I live in southern California where the big one is predicted to occur any time. I live in denial that the earth will quake near me, significantly, in my lifetime. However, I am still prepared. We have an emergency power generator for refrigeration and we have extra supplies of critical medications (insulin and other meds) as well as water and food supplies, just in case we lose power for an extended period of time and pharmacies are not open.

Earthquakes and tornadoes don't give you any advance warning. But if one strikes near your home or work, you can at least be prepared.

> ➤ Be sure to have enough supply of critical medications (insulin, pump supplies and syringes and other important medications).

➢ If you work farther than walking distance to your home, you might want to keep a supply of insulin and syringes as well as urgent medications at your workplace, in case the roads are impassable and you can't get home.

➢ Electricity may be interrupted so you may want to keep a hard copy of your medications and schedule, in case you need them.

➢ Keep a stash of food and water in your office and car, in case you are stranded.

Often, weather reports alert you about impending hurricanes and floods. If you hear warnings, please take these seriously and get prepared. Again, supplies, food, water, medications, and a printed version of your medical list could save your life.

A QUICK REVIEW OF KEY TOPICS:

• Natural Disasters: Earthquakes, Tornadoes, Hurricanes, and Floods

• If you live or travel to areas subject to natural disasters, **Be Prepared!**

• Keep:

  • Extra insulin and other critical medications and supplies near or with you,

  • A stash of food, snacks and water,

  • A hard copy of your medical lists in your wallet or purse or car. There might be a power outage and you can't use a computer to display/print your list. Having your important information on paper could be very useful.

PART 4: THE HOSPITAL VS. YOU

4.1   Hospital Management 101

4.2   The LIST: What you need to bring with you

4.3   Emergency Room-the ER

4.4   Your Hospital Stay

4.5   Your Pump, CGMS, Syringes, and Meters

46   Hospital Food: You are What You Eat

4.1 ~ Hospital Management 101

"A trip to the hospital is always a descent into the macabre.
I have never trusted a place with shiny floors."

~ Terry Tempest Williams, American author, conservationist and activist

---

KEY TOPICS

- Being in the hospital can be frightening
- Treat hospital staff with as much respect and kindness as you can muster

---

While I fear this will read like a primer from Psychology 101, I'll just jump right in.

HOSPITAL: n. [häs' pitl]: An institution providing medical and surgical treatment and nursing care for sick or injured people.

When you are a patient in a hospital, you are in a big, organized (or not so organized) corporation, with lots of departments and various skill levels, all orchestrated to administer care while you are ill.

There are a lot of different people delivering a lot of different services, each with differing levels of competence, kindness, expertise, and knowledge. You will have to quickly figure out who does what and how to get your needs met. To make it all the harder, shifts change and you can and will get new players every 12 hours (or more often).

So who are these players?

Doctors: That's why you are in the hospital. But remember, when you are in the hospital, you are on hospital time. Doctors visit at random times.

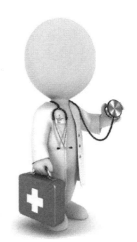

Be prepared. If you have questions or concerns, it is best to write them down. If you have to be out of the room/bed (to go to the bathroom or for a test), give your list of questions to your advocate (spouse, family member, friend, or at the least, your charge nurse), in case the doctor makes his appearance when you are not there.

Nurses: RNs (nurses who graduated from nursing programs at a college or university and have passed national licensing exams) are your primary path of communication to attending physicians (also known as "hospitalists"), surgeons and other members of your medical care team. These are the folks you want to establish a good relationship with, as best as you can. Indicate to them how you manage your health, show them your pump and blood glucose meter or CGMS, let them know at what time you need to take critical meds (and ask them to verify that they have the orders in your chart).

Nursing Assistants and Aides: These are the people who will make your life more comfortable. If you need a snack or an extra blanket or pillow, a back rub or a toothbrush, these are the ones who will help. Make friends. As one aide told me, he was the key to my getting released from the hospital, as he was the one who measured my input (fluids in) and my output (pee and poop). You won't be released until those are running smoothly.

Dieticians and Food Service Delivery: Dieticians are the ones who allocate the amount and type of food that has been specified by your doctor for your menus. Food trays are generally delivered on a regular schedule (times may vary):

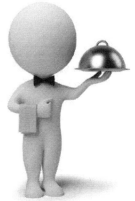

- ➤ Breakfast, with mid-day snack, around 7:30 AM
- ➤ Lunch, with mid-afternoon snack, around 11:30 AM
- ➤ Dinner, with bedtime snack, around 5:30 PM

If you don't like the type or quantity or options on your menu, you can always request a visit by the dietitian to discuss your meal plan and any modifications.

Other Servicers: Imaging techs, breathing specialists and the couriers (the ones who transport you via wheelchair) are all important parts of your care and recovery. Once again, make friends. Transporters can get you warm blankets as you are being moved and happy techs can just make the care much more pleasant.

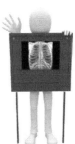

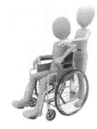

Remember, they are all people just doing a job. They have personal lives and stresses and pressures. Their job brings them in contact with cranky people. The more pleasant you and your advocates can be, the more they will go the extra mile to help. Even a smile just makes their jobs easier. Small talk can make them feel important and will also help you pass the time.

THE BEST ADVICE of ALL: Treat all of these people with the utmost kindness and respect. They have their hands full of patients, staff, and administration as well as their own personal pressures. But what you need from them is their *best* care of *you*. So treat them well and they will treat you as well as possible. Being in the hospital may be out of your control, but your attitude and treatment of others is up to you.

"I don't like that man. I must get to know him better."

~Abraham Lincoln, 16th President of the United States

NOSOCOMEPHOBIA: n. [no'-so-coe'-ma-fo'-be-a]: *The excessive fear of hospitals.*

According to Dr. Marc Siegal, associate professor at the New York University Medical Center, "It's perfectly understandable why many people feel the way they do about a hospital stay. You have control of your life, up until you're admitted to a hospital."

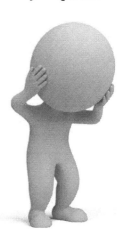

In fact, the late President Richard Nixon was known to have a fear of hospitals after refusing to get a treatment for a blood clot in 1974 saying, "If I go into the hospital, I'll never come out alive."

Having diabetes simply exacerbates the fear. We are taught that we must maintain control to stay alive. So going into the hospital, where we will not be in control, can scare us to death.

My mother was an avid Reader's Digest fan. Later, when I went to college I learned that reading the condensed version was considered cheating. Fortunately, she didn't subscribe to this view and read a series of articles entitled "I am Joe's (fill in the organ)". In this case, she had just read "I am Joe's Pancreas" and, given that I was skinny, thirsty, urinated frequently and had wounds from athletic activities that wouldn't heal, she was convinced that I had Diabetes. I was 11. It was 1964.

When she took me to the family doctor, he said she was a hypochondriac and that she was wrong about her diagnosis and should just take me home. I looked healthy enough — red cheeks, slender — and I was doing well in school. She was adamant that I be tested, arguing that my breath was "fruity smelling," and when it was revealed that my blood sugar was over 500, I was immediately hospitalized.

The doctor put me in a ward with older women, rather than the children's ward. I was purposely surrounded by amputee victims. They had lost toes, feet, and legs, and moaned all day and night. My doctor told me that this was my fate if I didn't EAT right.

I was there for a week. I learned to draw insulin (water, actually) and shoot into oranges and eventually my thighs. After returning home I gave myself my first injection without the aid of nurses before heading off to my 5th grade class. I injected the insulin through a dull needle and a glass syringe and then I looked up to see both of my parents with tears in their eyes. They were scared straight by the risk of complications and I was just beginning a very long and difficult journey.

Dale R., Type 1 diabetes for 48 years

Needless to say, being hospitalized scared me. NO, actually, it terrified me!

TERRIFIED: adj. [ter·ri·fied]

1. To be filled with terror; made deeply afraid.

2. To be menaced or threatened; intimidated.

Not only do I face the loss of control. I must place my fate and my life in the hands of strangers — often, overworked doctors, nurses and other staff members.

"Many patients go into a hospital on blind faith, because they think that whatever is being done to them is OK because it's a hospital," says Vincent Marchello, MD, medical director of Metropolitan Jewish Geriatric Center in New York City, and assistant clinical professor of medicine at Albert Einstein College of Medicine. "They shouldn't."

Now, that's scary! But there is a lot we can do, as diabetics, to be prepared and ensure the very best outcome possible.

A QUICK REVIEW OF KEY TOPICS:
HOSPITAL MANAGEMENT 101

- Acknowledge that being in the hospital can be a frightening prospect but realize that there are things you can do to make your experience successful.
- Treat hospital staff with as much respect and kindness as you can muster, realizing that they are overworked and very busy. The kinder you are to them, the better they will serve you.

4.2 ~ The LIST: What to Bring with You

"Organizing is what you do before you do something,
so that when you do it, it is not all mixed up."
~ A. A. Milne, English author

Here's a list of what you want to bring with you for your hospital stay:

➤ Your medication and allergy list

➤ Your medication schedule (when you take what and for what conditions)

➤ Your list of doctors

➤ Remember, you can be prepared by keeping your *The Savvy Diabetic: On The Go* workbook up-to-date and ready to go, available on www.TheSavvyDiabetic.com

What to include:

➤ Your insulin

➤ Any medications not routine (that the pharmacy may have difficulty getting. This could include sleeping aids, special injectables)

➤ Your insulin pump, including

✧ Cartridges

✧ Infusion sets

✧ IV Prep or whatever you use

➤ Your basal profile, printed, if you have it

➤ Syringe supplies

✧ Syringes

✧ Swabs

➤ If you use CGMS (continuous glucose monitoring system)

➤ Receiver

➤ Extra sensors

➤ IV Prep or whatever you use

➢ Hypofix or other tape to adhere your sensors or infusion sets

➢ Scissors to cut Hypofix

➢ Glucose Tabs (or whatever you prefer to use for low blood glucose)

➢ Batteries and/or Chargers

   ✧ For insulin pump

   ✧ For CGMS

➢ Cell phone

➢ iPad/Tablet/Laptop/Kindle

➢ Toiletries: Toothbrush, toothpaste, comb, hair products ~ things that will help you feel clean and human

➢ Robe and slippers

➢ Change of underwear

➢ Pillow, if that will help you sleep better

➢ Even a stuffed animal or a favorite framed photo

A QUICK REVIEW OF KEY TOPICS:
THE LIST: WHAT TO BRING WITH YOU

- Bring what you need to feel as comfortable, and at home, as possible.

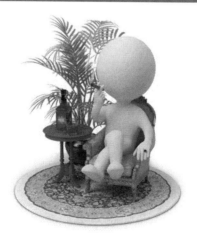

4.3 ~ Emergency Room — the ER

"First, the doctor told me the good news:
I was going to have a disease named after me."

~ Steve Martin, American actor, comedian, musician, author, playwright

---

KEY TOPICS

- Have someone you know stay with you in the ER.
- Bring your list of medications and physicians, along with food and quick sugar, your own blood glucose testing kit.
- Keep an emergency kit at home with supplies you might need in an emergency, with a note with extra items (insulin, chargers, batteries).
- Bring your own insulin and syringes as well as other medications.
- If you are very anxious, let the nursing staff know.
- Use your music player or book to help pass the waiting time.

EMERGENCY ROOM: n. Abbr. ER
[ih-mur-juhn-see room]: The section of a health care facility intended to provide rapid treatment for victims of sudden illness or trauma. Also now called the Emergency Department in many hospitals.

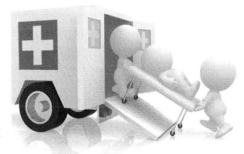

OK, you are headed to the ER. Probably not something you had planned or were hoping to do, and most likely, you are either injured or ill.

What's first?

➤ If at all possible, have someone you know (parent, spouse, sibling, friend, or adult child) with you. That person is your advocate, to help you communicate your issues and needs to the very busy hospital personnel.

You don't always have the choice, but whenever possible, have an advocate who is level-headed and calm, knows how to articulate your medical condition, is willing to help you ask questions, and can comprehend the answers.

It is a particularly overwhelming time during admission to the ER. You don't have much control and you are seeing a lot of personnel and being asked a lot of questions.

But if you are prepared, you will have your list of meds and physicians with you.

➤ Locate a source of food and quick sugar. Do you carry sugar with you? Bring it with you into the ER, in case your blood glucose starts to drop. If you don't have anything, ask your advocate or attending nurse or assistant to bring you some snacks and juice, just in case.

➤ Blood glucose testing supplies: Do not count on the ER staff to take the time to check your blood glucose. This is a stressful time, so you may want to check your own blood glucose, as needed.

Do you have enough supplies with you? If not, perhaps someone can bring them from your home. In that case, does someone have a key/access to your home and supplies? Is there a hide-a-key somewhere, for just these unexpected times? Do you keep a critical set of back up medications in the refrigerator?

➤ If you think you will be admitted to stay in the hospital, you will need chargers for your phone, CGMS, electronic tablet, etc. and batteries for your pump. It's a great idea to keep an emergency kit conveniently placed in your home with all the supplies you might need, along with a note with the extra items (insulin, chargers) that someone can pick up and bring to you.

➤ If you take insulin shots, having your own insulin and syringe will prevent you from waiting for a nurse to wait for a doctor's order to request a blood glucose test to then request insulin, which will have to be delivered from the pharmacy. All this could take well over two hours.

Of course, you will have to have permission from your attending physician and the cooperation of the nursing staff, so be sure to talk to them before taking your own insulin.

➤ If you need to take other meds at certain times, let the nursing staff know, clearly, what you need and when you need to take it. If you have the meds with you, check to see if you can take your own. If not, be persistent to get what you need when you need it. Again, this could take time, so if you need to take something at 6 pm, let them know well before that time and keep asking until they confirm that your medication has been ordered and will be delivered when you need it.

You could be in the ER for many LONG hours. After you are stabilized, you'll spend time waiting for the doctor, waiting for labs, waiting for CT's and X-rays, waiting for pain meds, waiting for admission to the hospital, waiting for a room/bed to become available, waiting for transportation, etc. That's a lot of waiting.

This can be so very frustrating but it is really just part of the system. So, as best as possible, RELAX! Know that you are in the best place to be while you are having a medical problem.

If being in the ER and not truly in charge causes you a lot of anxiety, let the nursing staff know. They may be able to give you something to calm you down or at least talk with you to allay your fears while you wait for answers, treatment, or pain relief.

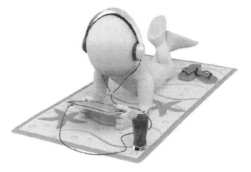

If you have an iPod/music player, you might want to pop in your earphones and allow yourself to become distracted while you settle in and wait.

"I've had a great time, but this wasn't it."
~ Groucho Marx, American comedian, and film/television star

A QUICK REVIEW OF KEY TOPICS
EMERGENCY ROOM—THE ER

- Have someone you know (parent, spouse, sibling, friend or adult child) with you.
- Bring your list of medications and physicians with you, along with food and quick sugar and your own blood glucose testing kit.
- Keep an emergency kit conveniently placed in your home with all the supplies you might need in an emergency, along with a note with the extra items (insulin, battery chargers, etc.). If you think you will be admitted to stay in the hospital, you will need chargers and batteries for your medical devices as well as your cell phone and digital tablets that someone can pick up and bring to you.
- If you take insulin shots, bring your own insulin and syringes. If you need to take other meds, bring them with you and check to see if you can take your own. If not, be persistent to get what you need when you need it.
- If being in the ER and not in control causes you a lot of anxiety, let the nursing staff know.
- If you have an iPod/music player, pop in your earphones and get distracted while you wait.

4.4.~ Your Hospital Stay

"According to hospital insurance codes,
there are 9 different ways you can be injured by turtles."
~ *Wall Street Journal*

KEY TOPICS

- Bring your advocate with you.
- Identify all the players on the hospital team, including doctors, nurses, nursing assistants, transport staff, technicians, lab folks, X-ray techs, volunteers, social workers, chaplain, billing personnel.
- Be as friendly as you possibly can, despite not feeling well, to get the best treatment and service.

You have now been admitted to the hospital and in your assigned room. What's next? You would do best to have your advocate with you as you settle in.

WHY IS THIS IMPORTANT AND WHAT IF I DON'T?

If you are in the hospital, you may be too sick or too injured to communicate well, and most likely:

- confined to your hospital bed,
- with an IV in your arm and,
- very tired.

Let your advocate listen in to what you are being told about your condition and what will be done. Allow your advocate to make sure you are comfortable, warm enough and settled in. At this point, your advocate can and will be your voice and your go-fetch person.

When you are moved to a hospital room, there is usually a board posted with names of the on-duty staff: charge nurse, attending nurse (that's the nurse assigned to your care), and nursing assistant. They will come in and introduce themselves during your orientation and assessment.

Here's your chance to establish yourself either you and/or your advocate.

1. Make sure the staff knows that you are either a Type 1 diabetic on insulin or a Type 2 diabetic on medication. Very often, as I mentioned earlier, if you say you are a diabetic, they may assume you have Type 2 diabetes, which requires completely different medications and attention.

2. Tell them how you administer your insulin.

   a. If you are on an insulin pump, show it to them and ask if they have any questions. (My experience has been that many, even in major metropolitan areas, have never seen an insulin pump. How is that possible? Makes me want to scream.) Unless you are incapable of managing your pump, your doctor will probably let you continue to use it, but it will be up to you to educate the rest of the staff.

   b. If you are wearing a CGMS, show them the sensor and the receiver. Explain how it gives you a constant reading, every one to five minutes. Very often, they will want to test your blood sugar with their old fashioned device.

TIP **Let 'em test you**	My experience has shown that it is best to let them do their own test and then show them that their readings are very close to those on your CGMS. Then, they may begin to trust your "gizmo" and ask you for your blood glucose readings instead using their own hospital glucose meter.

"Constant attention by a good nurse may be
just as important as a major operation by a surgeon."
~ Dag Hammarskjold, Swedish diplomat, economist and author

3. If you take other critical meds, let the nurses know what they are, when you take them, and what you will need from the staff.

4. Voice any concerns you have about your health, tests being ordered, or anything else that worries you.

5. The medical assistant will probably measure urine output, do vitals, get you snacks and whatever or whomever else you might need, including the nurse. The medical assistant is very important for your care and comfort.

6. Try to find out when your medical doctors might be coming by to see you. Their schedules are erratic and mostly unpredictable. It seems as if they show up when you are sleeping or when your advocate just went home. Very often, the nursing staff will estimate, based on their experience with your doctor, when he or she is likely to stop in. It is best to write down your list of concerns and questions so you are not caught by surprise.

> **TIP**
>
> **Catch the doctor before he/she leaves the floor**
>
> After the doctor sees you, he or she is often at the nurses' station for another 10 minutes, updating your chart. In case you have one more question, your doctor might still be on the floor.

7. You will be wheeled out of your room by orderlies for tests and x-rays. A smile or a friendly word always helps. Don't forget to ask for the extra warm blanket to keep you snug and warm.

8. If you are in the hospital long enough (more than three days), you may get a visit from a social worker or chaplain. Feel free to discuss your anxieties and needs with the social worker or chaplain who will try to help. You will also probably get visits from candy striper volunteers or book cart volunteers.

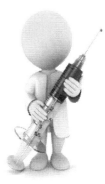

9. Usually there will be a lot of lab work done. The lab techs come in very early (often 4:00 to 5:00 AM).

TIP	If you know you have one arm with a better vein, remember to tell them. If you know what works best for the draw (drinking fluids, warm compress, letting your arm dangle) or what you hate (no blood drawn from your wrist), let them know, each and every time.
Drawing blood	

10. Business office personnel may come to visit you, to discuss your medical insurance coverage. Remember, they are just doing their job to ensure that the hospital gets reimbursed and the staff gets paid for their work.

"It's no longer a question of staying healthy;
it's a question of finding a sickness you like."

~ *Jackie Mason, American stand-up comedian*

A Quick Review of Key Topics:
Your Hospital Stay

- This is the time to rely on your advocate. If at all possible, have your advocate with you in the emergency room.
- Identify all the players on the hospital roster:
  - Doctors
  - Nurses
  - Nursing Assistants
  - Transport Staff
  - Medical Technicians
  - Lab Phlebotomists (those who draw your blood)
  - X-ray Technicians
  - Volunteers (candy stripers, chaplain)
  - Business Office Personnel
- Be as friendly as you possibly can, despite the fact that you are not feeling well, maybe are in pain, and are simply exhausted.

4.5 ~ What about your Insulin Pump, CGMS, Syringes and Meters?

"Any sufficiently advanced technology
is indistinguishable from magic."
~ *Arthur C. Clarke, British science fiction author, inventor and futurist*

KEY TOPICS

- Be prepared to explain your knowledge, and use of, your insulin pump or syringes with insulin.
- Expect curiosity about your CGMS and even your insulin pump.
- Keep your own meter and strips with you.
- Put your name and contact information on your devices.
- Where to wear your devices.

Insulin Pump: n [in-suh-lin puhmp]: a medical device used for the administration of insulin in the treatment of diabetes, also known as continuous subcutaneous insulin infusion therapy.

Believe it or not, many hospital personnel (doctors, nurses and assistants) have never seen an insulin pump. Hard to believe, isn't it? It's true.

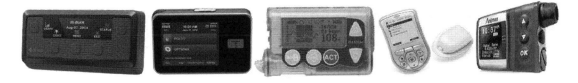

Many ER personnel are trained to pull your pump off and institute their sliding scale for insulin dosing, which may have nothing to do with your needs!

If you are alert and capable, if at all possible, try to keep your pump connected and running. Discuss the use of your pump with the charge nurse and the attending physician and anesthesiologist. Explain your insulin profile. Show them that you can suspend the insulin delivery, if necessary. Very often, once they understand that you know how to manage your insulin delivery, they will allow you to use it, as long as they can monitor your blood glucose levels.

If you are scheduled for surgery, discuss your pump with your surgeon, the physician who will manage your diabetes, and the anesthesiologist. Show them how to disconnect and/or shut off the pump. Once they are comfortable with the pump, they will, most likely, allow you to stay connected.

Continuous Glucose Monitoring System (CGMS): n. [see jee em es]: an FDA-approved device that records blood sugar levels throughout the day and night.

I can almost guarantee you that most hospital staffers have not even heard of a continuous glucose monitoring system (CGMS). And some will be fascinated!

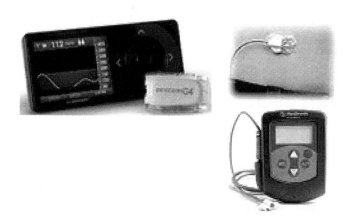

This is your opportunity, if you feel well enough, to educate them about this amazing technology and how it can help them to help you. I've found that after they test my blood glucose with their outdated blood glucose machines and compare the readings with your CGMS, they will stop testing you and simply ask you what your "little doohickey" says!

Syringes, Insulin and Meters

If you are still using syringes or pen needles, be sure to bring your own syringes, or pen needles and insulin, with you to the hospital. You do not want to have to wait for a nurse to contact a doctor for your regular insulin.

It is also helpful to bring your own personal blood glucose testing meter and supplies with you. The nurses may insist that they test your blood glucose with their clunky equipment. But if you can show them that your readings are the same as they are getting, they may let you test for yourself, and show them or tell them the results.

"Laughter is the best medicine — unless you're diabetic,
then insulin comes pretty high on the list."

~ *Jasper Carrott, English comedian, actor, television personality*

It's Mine! Give it a label

Put a label with your name and contact information, in case you lose or leave your insulin pump remote or CGMS receiver. Unless someone knows how to return it, you could be faced with buying a replacement.

I learned this lesson the stressful way. I was sitting in the theater, enjoying a wonderful play, actually not thinking about diabetes for a while. After the standing ovation, we gathered our coats and made our way up the aisle and out to our car.

That's when I noticed. My CGMS receiver was GONE! Not in my pocket (where I usually keep it), not tucked away in my bra and not in my purse. It had fallen out of my pocket and I didn't hear it drop to the floor. My husband ran back in to the theater and found an usher.

Together, they searched the aisles. No CGMS receiver! My husband went to the business office and AHA, it was there! Someone had kindly turned it in.

But then he was asked to identify it. In the flurry of the search, he had to remember the brand of CGMS and what it looked like. Wow, was he stressed out!

Now there is a label on the back with my cell phone number and the word REWARD.

WHY IS THIS IMPORTANT AND WHAT IF I DON'T?

- Always put a label on your CGMS, meter and insulin pump remote device (PDM or remote controller), with your name and contact information.
- If you should lose any of these, someone can actually return your essential equipment back to you.
- By the way, this is also a great idea for your cell phone, iPad, camera and other valuable electronic devices.

Where to carry your devices?I was skipping over this topic until one of my editors, a non-diabetic friend, asked me about the description of hiding my pump in my bra. She looked baffled. She asked, "Well, where do men wear their pumps?" So I thought I would quickly describe some options for stowing your pump, syringes and insulin, remote controllers, and CGMS receivers.

The first and most obvious place is in your pocket. Of course, that's simple enough. But if you are carrying your wallet and your sunglasses, you may run out of pocket room in your pants or shirt pocket.

You can stick your pump or CGMS receiver in your bra or your underpants. But this comes with warnings:

Be aware when you undress that your device can drop to the floor.

Check for loose or exposed tubing, which can easily get caught on knobs and door handles.

You can stick the pump in your sock. There are even socks with zippers to hold your pump or remote.

There are fanny packs and stretchy thigh bands in a variety of colors and styles. You can have one to match every outfit.

You will find some resources in the Appendix where you can order these nifty products. There is even a YouTube video called Where to Wear the Insulin Pump!

A QUICK REVIEW OF KEY POINTS: INSULIN PUMP, CGMS, SYRINGES AND METERS

- Be prepared to explain your knowledge and use of your insulin pump or syringes with insulin. Ask to be allowed to use the system (insulin delivery, testing and dosing) you know works for you.
- Expect curiosity about your CGMS. Nurses, nursing students, nursing assistants and even some doctors may not have seen the newest technology
- Keep your own meter and strips with you, so that you may test whenever you want, not on their schedule.
- Label your medical electronics with your name and contact information, in case it gets misplaced.
- Get creative with where you wear your medical devices.

4.6 ~ Hospital Food: You Are What You Eat

"I never worry about diets.
The only carrots that interest me
are the number you get in a diamond."

~ Mae West, American actress, singer, playwright, and sex symbol

---

KEY TOPICS

- If at all possible, specify/request an OPEN DIET.
- Keep glucose tabs near you.
- Feel free to request a visit from the dietician.

Hospital food conjures up horror stories and comedy routines, and a lot of what you know or have heard is true.

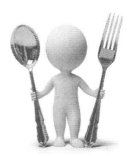

1. If you like to have control (there's that word again) over what you order and what is delivered to you, ask your doctor to specify Open Diet. If your doctor calls for Diabetic Diet, you will get a certain number of calories, designed for an American Medical Association Type 2 diabetes diet, including carbs you may not want or food you won't eat.

2. If there are special snacks or foods that you prefer, you can always bring them in with you or have someone bring them, unless you are on a restricted diet.

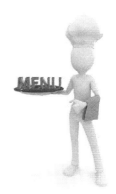

3. If there is a form of glucose that you prefer to use for low blood glucose, bring that with you and keep it near you. It's better to use what you know works and not wait for a busy assistant to get you juice, or worse, crackers and cheese for low blood sugar!

Bottom line: Unless your diet is restricted for medical reasons, it is always easier to maintain control of your diabetes with food ad meds that you know.

"The first law of dietetics seems to be:
if it tastes good, it's bad for you."

~ Isaac Asimov, American author and professor of biochemistry

---

A QUICK REVIEW OF KEY TOPICS:
YOU ARE WHAT YOU EAT

- If at all possible, specify/request an OPEN DIET, which allows you to choose the foods and the amounts you usually eat.
- Keep glucose tablets (or whatever you use for low blood glucose episodes) in your nightstand, next to your bed.
- If you have any questions or special needs (vegetarian or kosher or other restrictions), you may always request a visit from the dietician.

Part 5: Travel Near and Far

5.1   Around Town and Short Trips

    ✧ Wear your medical ID tag

    ✧ Keep snacks and fast glucose handy

    ✧ Sources of quick sugar

    ✧ Your up-to-date lists

5.2   Faraway Journeys

    ✧ Security check points and TSA rules

    ✧ Carry a travel letter

    ✧ Pack snacks and sugar

    ✧ Bring back up supplies

    ✧ Pack your list

    ✧ Conversions and power adapters

5.1 ~ Around Town and Short Trips

"When you come to a fork in the road...take it."

~ Yogi Berra, former American League Baseball player and manager

---

KEY TOPICS

- Wear a medical ID tag.
- Keep snacks and ready glucose with you.
- Carry your up-to-date lists of medications, emergency contacts, and doctors.
- Carry back up syringes and insulin, as well as insulin pump supplies, just in case.
- Inexpensive generic blood glucose meters and strips are available from pharmacies.
- Emergency RX can be filled at nation-wide pharmacy chains.
- Wear glasses or contact: bring a back-up pair and Rx for your correction.
- How to find medical help, away from home.

TRAV·EL: n. [trav-l]: To go from one place to another, as on a trip; journey.m

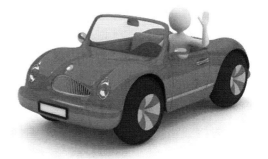

Wear Your Medical ID Tag, Always

You should always wear a tag that identifies you as diabetic and who to call in case of an emergency.

ID tags have become much more fashionable than when I was first diagnosed and all I could get was clunky stainless steel bracelet.

WHY IS THIS IMPORTANT AND WHAT IF I DON'T

Emergencies can happen, without warning.

• Another car can rear-end your car

• Your blood glucose levels might suddenly drop

• You could get hit by a meteor

• Or any other unforeseen event, where you are unable to speak clearly or may indeed be unconscious.

You want emergency responders to know your medical conditions immediately. They are trained to look for medical ID tags.

Wear one. It speaks for you when you can't.

There are several organizations that offer a variety of alert tags, including:Medic Alert Foundation, which offers to store your medical information as well as your list of emergency contacts and doctors in their database, accessible via an 800 number.

Your local pharmacy sells basic medical ID tags as well as tags that may be personalized.

Lauren's Hope (www.LaurensHope.com) offers a large selection of fashion medical ID jewelry, for men, women, and kids.

RoadID: "It's Who I Am" (www.RoadID.com) sells durable, rugged, athletic, fashionable identification gear, including bands for your wrist, ankle, or shoe.

CapeCodEMR (www.capecodemr.com) offers emergency medical record USB devices, in a variety of formats.

Now there is no excuse. Wear your medical ID tag proudly and be safe.

Snacks and Glucose

It is always wise to carry a source of fast-acting glucose as well as snacks with you, either in your briefcase, handbag or stashed in your car.

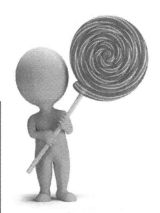

> ### WHY IS THIS IMPORTANT AND WHAT IF I DON'T?
>
> If you can't eat as you planned, it is helpful to have a snack to hold you over until food arrives.
>
> Your blood glucose can drop suddenly from:
>
> - Exercise
> - Miscalculating the carbs in a meal
> - Stress
> - Delays in getting your meal
> - Or for no obvious reason
>
> If you carry your own glucose, you'll be able to quickly correct the low blood glucose.

Some Suggested Sources of Quick Sugar

➢ Glucose tablets

➢ Dried fruit bars

➢ Juice

➢ Lifesavers, jelly beans or any other non-chocolate, non-melting candy

Keep your Up-To-Date Lists with you

We've already covered this. Be sure to keep your updated list of medications, prescriptions, emergency contacts and doctors, either in printed form or on a flash drive, just in case.

Insulin Pumps, Rx's and Meters, Away from Home

What do you do if you are away from home and:

➢ You can't find your meter?

➢ You run out of testing strips?

➢ Your only bottle of insulin breaks?

➢ You lose or run out of a prescription medication?

➢ Your insulin pump fails?

If your blood glucose meter breaks or you left it at home, you can go to any pharmacy in one of the big box stores (Walmart, CostCo, Target, Walgreens) and buy a new meter which usually comes with a sample size bottle of 10 test strips.

TIP Generic Meters	These stores also sell generic, no-brand inexpensive meters along with low-price generic test strips. They work well and will solve your problem quickly.

If your insulin bottle breaks or freezes and you use insulin that requires a prescription (Novolog and Humalog requires a doctor's Rx), ask your healthcare provider to give you a current Rx on his Rx pad or letterhead, which you can take to any pharmacy, to replace your bottle of insulin.

If you lose or run out of a prescription medication, there could be a quick fix for this too.

TIP
Keep Important RX's at Big Box Store Pharmacies

Even if you usually purchase your prescription drugs at a local pharmacy or via mail-order, you could also keep some of your critical prescriptions on file at one of the larger pharmacy retailers (Target, Costco, Walmart, RiteAid, CVS, Walgreens, etc.). If you find you suddenly need to refill one of your important prescriptions, you can walk into any of these stores, nationwide, and they will have your insurance information and be able to fill your Rx, in a pinch

TIP
Carry a Loaner Insulin Pump

Many insulin pump companies will lend you a back-up pump during your travel, just in case. If they don't have that policy, you might be able to find someone in a support group or your physician's office who will lend you a pump for the duration of your travel.

Eyeglasses: Back Up Pair and Rx

Do you wear glasses for distance or for reading? What happens if they break or you lose them? How will you fill a syringe, use your pump or read your CGMS receiver or blood glucose meter read-out?

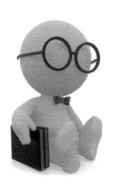

I always travel with a second pair of my prescription glasses (usually an older pair, maybe not with the most current prescription but close enough), as well as the correction prescription from my optometrist. If you suddenly don't have your glasses, you can take the Rx to any optical shop that offers quick turnaround service.

TIP	
Your eyeglasses	If you really need your glasses to see distance or close-up, be sure to carry a back-up pair of glasses and your optometrist's prescription for your necessary correction.

Need a doctor on the road?

What if you are several miles away from home and suddenly become sick, develop a high fever or other serious symptoms? What if you are in an accident? What if you trip and break a bone? There is no time to get home to your regular doctors and you need a medical team fast.

First, and most obviously, you can always go to the nearest emergency room. Of course, after having read this complete survival guide, you will have your medical information on a flash drive or hard copy, with you.

But then, what if you need surgery or further medical care? Here are some tips for finding the best medical care away from home.

➤ If you are visiting friends or know people (colleagues, old college friends, etc.) where you need help, call them for referrals and assistance in getting in to seek the medical help you need.

- ➤ If you are a member of a service organization (Rotary International, Kiwanis, Lions Club, etc.), contact any member of the local chapter and ask for help.
- ➤ Contact the local chapters of JDRF or American Diabetes Association for the support group whose members may readily reach you to help you.
- ➤ Talk to the pharmacist at the local drugstore for a referral. They tend to know who the best doctors are in the area.
- ➤ If you are experiencing a diabetes-related emergency, try to contact the local sales representatives for the diabetes products you use. Again, they most likely know the endocrinologists in the area as well as other specialists.

Remember, if you are having an emergency away from home, reach out to people and organizations that may be able to hook you up to the best care in town.

"In a day if you don't come across any problems, you can be sure
that you are travelling in a wrong way."
~ *Swami Vivekanand, Indian Hindu monk and disciple of Ramakrishna*

A QUICK REVIEW OF KEY TOPICS:
AROUND TOWN AND SHORT TRIPS

- Wear a medical ID tag, always.
- Keep snacks and ready glucose with you.
- Carry your up-to-date lists of medications, emergency contacts, and doctors in hard copy or on a flash drive.
- Keep back up syringes and insulin, as well as insulin pump supplies, with you, just in case.
- Inexpensive generic blood glucose meters and strips are available
- from large chain pharmacies. There has been question about their absolute accuracy, but they are better than having no meter at all.
- Emergency prescriptions can be filled at nation-wide pharmacy chains, as long as your Rx is on file.
- Carry a second pair of your prescription glasses as well as an Rx with your vision correction.
- If you do have an emergency and need to find the best medical doctor in a pinch, contact friends, business associates, service organizations, JDRF or ADA, pharmacists or sales representatives for the best referrals.

5.2 ~ Faraway Journeys

"Boy, those French. They have a different word for everything."

~ Steve Martin, American humorist

KEY TOPICS

- Wear a medical ID tag.
- Be aware of security and TSA rules, carry prescriptions for medications and supplies, and bring lists of medications, emergency and medical contacts.
- Keep snacks and ready-glucose with you.
- Keep a back-up supply of everything at home.
- Be prepared for conversions, including power adapters.

Is your slogan: Have insulin (and supplies), will travel?

Is your lifestyle motto: "On the road again," or "I'm outta here"?

Is it that simple, for a person with diabetes to get up and go?

The answer is yes, as long as you are prepared.

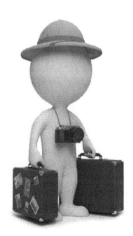

Here are some tips that will make you safe and able when you are away from home, whether it is for a few hours away or on the other side of the world.

Security Check Points and TSA rules

The Transportation Security Administration regulates the security of traveling in the U.S. Before you fly somewhere, within the U.S. or internationally, learn the rules for transporting medications and supplies so that you will be not be surprised during your travel. If travelling during high alert times, be aware that regulations may become more stringent. Remember, insulin is a fluid and syringes, insulin pumps, and CGMS are devices that may cause concern at the gate.

While it is safe to put your insulin, insulin pump, CGMS receiver, and medicines through the x-ray devices, the alarms may trigger with your pump, meter and receiver. Whenever I go through security screening, I disconnect my pump and place it, my meter, and my CGMS receiver in the plastic bins. I usually also tell the gate agent that I wear an insulin pump because I am diabetic. Remember, they are just doing their job so the more helpful you are, the easier you will sail through the checkpoints.

> *If you are a frequent traveler, check out being certified for TSA-Pre.*
>
> *You go through a short, dedicated line, metal detector only, and do not have to remove any liquids, take off shoes, take off jacket, or remove computer during screening. The metal detector doesn't even see the Omnipod, since it isn't metal, so no hand swabbing or pat down.*
>
> *For more information see: http://www.tsa.gov/tsa-precheck.*
>
> *It's a terrific stress and time saver, if you travel a lot.. You have to go to a major airport for the interview and fingerprinting.*
>
> Barbara G., Type 1.5, LADA for 11 years

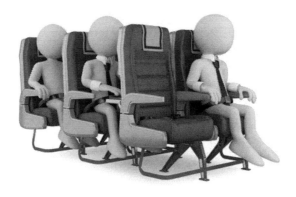

If you are travelling in a foreign country, you could also write down the words in their native language: "I have diabetes. I wear an insulin pump. I carry syringes to take insulin, my medication. I wear a device to monitor my blood glucose."

For some commonly traveled countries, find this phrase translated in Section 9.6.

> *To anyone about to travel, my advice is just to bring lots of extra supplies and not to worry about it! In the past 8 years I've been to the Bahamas, Belize, Cambodia, Canada, Chile, China, Costa Rica, Easter Island, Egypt, El Salvador, England, France, Hong Kong, India, Italy, Kenya, Mexico, Nicaragua, Peru, United Arab Emirates, and Vietnam not to mention many places with the U.S.*
>
> *Yes, I've been pulled aside for special screening many places but nothing has ever caused me a major delay. Issues have all been taken care of within ten minutes or less. If I get pulled aside by people who don't speak English, which was the case often in China, before I go into a separate room with airport screening officials, I find someone in security who speaks English to go in with me. There has always been someone who is willing to help!*
>
> *Yes, I've been asked to remove my Pod (Omnipod), but after explaining why I can't, they swab it and let me leave it on. I carry a doctor's note just in case. But if you don't have one I wouldn't worry about that either, as when I showed it in the United Arab Emirates and China, they could care less about it since it's written in English and not in Arabic/Mandarin.*
>
> Casey O., Type 1 diabetes for 20 years

Carry a travel letter from your doctor, and labels for supplies and meds

FI have never needed to use this, but I carry an Rx from my doctor for syringes and insulin, just in case. Better to err on the safe side, in case you need help. Keep all your supplies (meters, strips, sensors, pump supplies, insulin, and glucagon) with you in your carry-on luggage.

> *No one has ever questioned the port sticking out of me. (Maybe they think it is some cool new piercing in your stomach?). Once I get my bag back, I just reattach the pump. I have never been questioned about my pills or even both back up syringes and pump supplies in my carry on.*
>
> *I flew recently and the TSA was more concerned about a small crystal clock my dad had given me to take home than my medical stuff I tried flying with a doctor's note once and no one even asked about it.*
>
> Laurie D., Type 1 diabetes

Carry-on vs. checked bags

Be sure to keep all your essential medications, supplies and medical equipment in your carry-on bag. On a recent trip, the airline lost my checked suitcase. Fortunately, it was on the flight home, and still, all my back-up supplies and extra pump were in my carry-on. The airline found my baggage the next day, in Hawaii. They delivered it to my home 24 hours after my flight home. I'm just glad it was on the homebound portion of my vacation and that my important medications and supplies were with me.

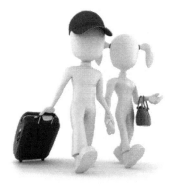

Pack snacks and low blood glucose treats or glucose tabs

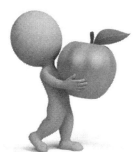

Flights and food service can be delayed. For both short and longer flights and travel, bring more food. Carry whatever you might need for low blood glucose episodes. You don't want to have to wait for a busy flight attendant or food service employee. In the instance that there are no more snacks available on your flight, you'll be fine.

Chargers and power adapters

If you require chargers for your pump or CGMS, check on the power specifications for your travel destination. You might need to bring AC power adapters with you.

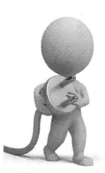

Back-up supplies

When you are traveling, especially out of the country, leave a FedEx box of supplies (including an extra pump, if you have it, CGMS supplies, and any hard to get medications) with a friend or in your home, refrigerated for the meds that need that. Just in case you lose your supplies and/or your reserves, someone should have a replacement or access to a replacement, ready to ship. Don't forget to include a second cell phone charger and charger for your CGMS.

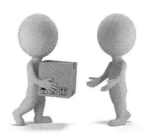

With the FedEx box ready to go, you can have your friend send it to a major hotel nearest you. Western hotels are used to receiving packages for guests and the delivery is more certain to a well-known hotel.

Back to Basics — your list

Pack your list of medications and allergies, emergency contacts, and medical team. Keep a copy in your luggage, one in your wallet and one on a flash drive. You can also keep copies of the information in the cloud, if you are technologically savvy.

Again, this means:

➤ List of all your medications and supplements (indicate dosages, how much, and when you take each) and allergies,

➤ Detail the condition for what you take each medication (including whether it is critical or optional),

➤ List your doctors, their contact information and specialty,

➤ Make a copy of your insurance card(s) and driver's license,

➤ Identify any significant members of your support system (spouse, children, and friends) and their contact information,

➤ Bring your list of items you will need if you are hospitalized.

Conversions

Blood Glucose:

➤ Whereas, in the U.S., we usually use mg/dl when measuring blood glucose, much of the world uses mmol/l.

➤ It's always a great idea to know how to convert from mg/dl to mmol/l and vice-a-versa in case you need medical help or are hospitalized in a foreign country.

➤ You can copy the chart in Part Nine: Appendix 9.5 and carry it with your medical lists and passport.

➤ Keep this conversion formula below with you as well as on a flash drive, just in case.

➤ To calculate:

✧ To convert mmol/l of glucose to mg/dl, multiply by 18

✧ To convert mg/dl of glucose to mmol/l, divide by 18 or multiply by 0.055

Temperature:

You'll find a conversion chart in Part Nine: Appendix 9.7 to help you quickly convert between Celsius and Fahrenheit.

When I was 15, I traveled with a high school group to spend a summer in France. I was actually doing very well in managing my diabetes but then I got the flu! I had to communicate with the infirmary doctor as best as I could. I remember being so frightened when they took my temperature it was 39! I did not know the conversion from Celsius to Fahrenheit so I didn't know how sick I was.

If you love math, here is the pen and paper method of conversion:

Temp C = (5 divided by 9) multiplied by (Temp F - 32)

OR

Temp F = (9 divided by 5) multiplied by Temp C + 32

Better yet, if you have a cell phone or computer tablet with you, you might want to install an application for conversion

Here are just a few adventures about traveling with diabetes.

The way I travel, as a diabetic, changed after 9/11. I was flying from Athens, Greece, through Frankfurt, Germany, to California. At Frankfurt Airport, even though it was just a lay-over, we were all placed in a room waiting to go through security again. Tensions were high after the shocking events from just a week before, so everyone understood and patiently waited to be directed to go through security once more.

When it was my turn, the airport security officer waved his wand around me. The wand went off on my left side. I told the officer, "Don't worry, I am wearing an insulin pump." He asked me to wait on the side so that a female officer could pat me down. When the female officer patted me down, she stopped when she felt my pump. The look of shock on her face, with eyes bulging out, I needed to reassure her, and quickly. "It's OK, it's my insulin pump. I'm diabetic." She acted like she had heard of such a thing but asked me what it looked like and if she could see it. I showed it to her in a back room and she reluctantly gave a nod of approval.

Since then, I've learned that my pump sets off the alarm at most airport security gates. To prevent a pat-down and personal screening, I just remove my pump before I get to the security gates and place it in my bag so that it goes through the x-ray machine with the rest of my belongings. Then I put it back on after I go through the security gates.

I also wear my infusion set in the front of my body. After a flight, the infusion will inevitably get compromised if I wear it on my bottom or back-side. At my destination, then I can move it to my bottom so that I can wear a bathing suit!

I know that all large airlines carry syringes on their planes. If you have insulin and no syringes, you can ask to use one. Warning ~ the syringes are huge, not like the tiny ones that we use for insulin shots. Lufthansa carries a first aid kit with syringes and the stewardess said that all planes do for these situations

Julianna A., Type 1 diabetes for 25 years

The CAT Scan Souvenir: Back in my college days, I attended a university study trip to Guadalajara, Mexico, and came back with lots of great souvenirs, including a CAT scan of my brain. I had fallen unconscious from hypoglycemia while sleeping, and my Mexican host family was vigilant enough to take me quickly to the local Hospital Mexico-Americano, where the doctors decided that an IV of glucose wasn't enough. They placed me in a CAT scan device and produced multiple images of my brain.

This wasn't quite the set of photos my parents were hoping for; however, thousands of dollars later, they were glad my brain and I survived. After the incident, I was relieved to know that my host family and my parents were both willing to let me stay in Mexico to finish my trip and education.

Sandra S., Type 1 diabetes for 26 years

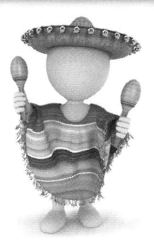

"NOT I — NOT ANYONE else, can travel that road for you.
You must travel it for yourself"

~*Walt Whitman, American poet, essayist and journalist*

A QUICK REVEIW OF KEY TOPICS
FARAWAY JOURNEYS

- Wear a medical ID tag always.
- Be aware of security and TSA rules; carry prescriptions for medications and supplies, and bring lists of medications, emergency and medical contacts. Carry a doctor's letter (with Rx) and labels from meds and supplies.
- Bring your medications and supplies in your carry-on luggage. Your checked luggage could be delayed or lost. You can always buy extra clothes but it's much harder to replace medications and supplies.
- Keep snacks and ready glucose with you, no in your checked luggage, but rather where you can get to them easily.
- Keep a back-up supply of everthing at home, in a packing box, in case you need someone to ship you supplies on the other side of the world.
- Know the power requirements for your destination and bring the appropriate adapters with you. Be prepared for conversions (between mmol/l to mg/dl and Centigrade to Fahrenheit.

PART 6: LIFESTYLE ISSUES

6.1   Having Babies or Not?

6.2   Spouses, Partners, Families and Friends

    ✧ A diabetic child in the family

    ✧ Young adult with diabetes

    ✧ Spouses and partners and friends

    ✧ How to communicate

    ✧ Reach out to resources

6.1 ~ Having Babies or Not?

"Having a child is surely the most beautifully irrational act
that two people in love can commit."

Bill Cosby, American comedian, actor, author, educator

KEY TOPICS

- Carefully consider your decision to have a baby.
- Babies of diabetic mothers can be delivered healthy and happy.
- Be prepared to work hard to deliver a healthy baby.

When I was just a teenager, I was told that I could never have children. (I was also told I could never be a pilot or other professions.) Indeed, Dr. Dolger, whom I mentioned earlier, wrote the following in his book, *How to Live with Diabetes*, copyright 1958:

"One of the most unusual aspects of the disease is the apparent link to marriage and motherhood. The highest number of deaths from diabetes is among married women — and this includes widows and divorcees. The death rate among married women is almost twice as great as among single women.

The married man is far less susceptible than the married woman. For him, the wedded state acts as a protection, and his death rate from diabetes is lower than that of bachelors, widowers, or divorces.

Why should women be more susceptible to diabetes than men, and married women more than single women? Motherhood seems to be the reason. The woman with more children is more susceptible than the women with fewer children. The more pregnancies a women undergoes, the greater is the possibility that she will become diabetic."

The message I got during my teen years was that pregnancy was extremely difficult and dangerous for a Type 1 diabetic and could lead to severe complications and even death, not only for me, but for the child. That scared me! It also scared my mom.

I was also frightened about having a child who might develop diabetes, and that just didn't feel fair. Then there was the 1989 movie, Steel Magnolias, in which the character, Shelby, a Type 1 diabetic, got pregnant, developed kidney failure and died. That just added to my fears.

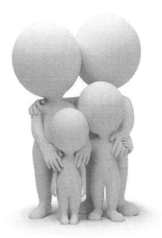

For every diabetic who chose not to have a baby, there are diabetics who made the decision to have a baby. Everyone has a different story and different motivation.

The process of giving birth to a healthy child is rigorous. Since I chose not to have children, I am relying on my diabetic friends, and diabetes literature for the best tips:

> *I decided not to have kids because I would worry too much about complications for a baby if things didn't go well for me during the pregnancy. Also, I've always had a very weak immune system (even before getting diabetes) and get sick often, which I worried would interfere with my ability to raise a kid the way I ideally think it should be done.*
>
> *Just because I have diabetes doesn't mean my kid will, but if my kid did (get diabetes), it would stress me out beyond belief! I couldn't imagine chasing after little ones trying to test their blood glucose. Instead, I get to enjoy my three nephews and then send them home when I'm sick!*
>
> Casey O., Type 1 diabetes for over 15 years

For me, knowing that having diabetes does not necessarily mean that the child will be diabetic helped me in making the decision. I did everything I was told to do, by the book, to make sure that he had the healthiest gestation I could give him. For me, it essentially was a more regimented meal plan and I had to eat more than I ever used to, per doctor's orders. But I am really good at doing what I am told so I would not say it was difficult.

In fact, I loved every part of being pregnant and will do it again, if it is meant to be.

Shelly R., Type 1 diabetes for over 20 years and a new mom

I made the choice not to have children. But in 1988, while my diabetes was in poor control, I inadvertently got pregnant. Before I even knew that I was pregnant, I had lost 50% of my kidney function and was hospitalized in critical condition. I saw several high risk pregnancy specialists and nephrologists.

I ended up losing the pregnancy, but not the kidney failure. I subsequently had tubal ligation which alleviated future pregnancy fears.

Sharon R., Type 1 diabetes for over 40 years

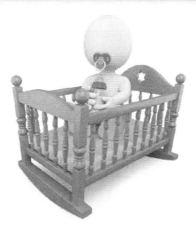

When I became diabetic at 24, I was told I would never have babies because diabetic women lost their babies in the 3rd trimester and/or the pregnancy might kill me.

Hmmm. I wanted to have a baby, and when I married my husband, we decided to have one child (he already had two). I was 34. It was my OB/GYN who convinced me that it was time to get my blood sugars under control and to start trying. Being high risk because of the diabetes, I was chronologically "older" than my age—around 40, he said—(which was considered pretty old, then, to have a baby).

It was a long and difficult pregnancy only in that I tested constantly and gave myself many, many shots per day. I knew that the baby was on the bigger side but I was told there was no reason that I shouldn't be able to deliver vaginally. As it turned out, having nothing to do with that, she was wrapped around the umbilical cord and I had to have an emergency caesarian section. She weighed 9 lbs, 2 ozs.

Charlotte, my baby, had to go into the ICU to monitor her blood sugars (in the womb, babies metabolize higher blood sugars than babies of non-diabetics). I contracted a horrible staph infection and was in the hospital for 10 days. Mike fed her before I did (I couldn't hold her with a high fever and an infection).

Her scores were all perfect, she is now a non-diabetic 24 year-old and, to date, has been very healthy. She refuses to get checked for the genetic markers for diabetes, which I, of course, wish she would.

PS—I didn't have to take insulin for almost a week after Charlotte was born. It was amazing!

Linda R., Type 1 diabetes over 30 years

This is Shelby's story. (No, not the same Shelby as in Steel Magnolias!)

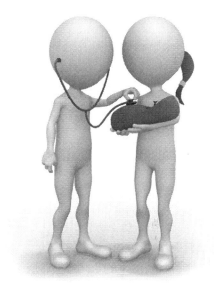

Since I had never had "woman" issues I just went to my GP for my yearly pap smears. When I decided to get pregnant, I was referred to a couple of OB/Gyn's. I interviewed them and decided to go with Dr. F. (she was okay and was recommended by my endocrinologist). With my age of 37 and my medical background, she recommended I find a high-risk OB. Again, I interviewed a couple of doctors, and went with Dr. P, because he only dealt with high-risk patients, he had a fabulous reputation, his office was in the parking lot of the hospital near my home (if anything went wrong during an appointment, I could be wheeled to the hospital straight away, which did happen). Lastly, there was a children's hospital on the 5th floor of the hospital in case my baby had to stay in the NICU.

During my first pregnancy, I continued to see both doctors. They would battle over what my dosages should be and what meds I should take. It also meant more doctors' appointments. I was like a child between fighting parents. With my second pregnancy, I only saw Dr. P and it was so much easier. My levels were good and there were fewer appointments. Because Dr. P. was very familiar with diabetic patients, I felt comfortable with the choices he made with my care.

Dr. P. was very strict. I had to record everything I ate and send the log to him twice a week. If he saw anything he didn't like, he would call me to change my basal or bolus rate. I also saw him every other week and I got an ultrasound every time. He wanted to monitor the baby's process every step of the way. Dr. P.'s staff was tiny and I knew everyone there and they knew me. I had email addresses, and I even had Dr. P.'s phone number when he went on vacation toward the end of my pregnancy. All the reasons I picked Dr. P. made things easier: his knowledge and reputation, his staff and location. He was a rock star. I wouldn't change a thing.

Birthing location was very important to me. I planned that my babies could stay in the NICU and I wanted a place that could accommodate them. The hospital I chose was smaller than some in the area. I didn't want my babies or me to get lost in the shuffle.

Both babies were in the NICU. The first time we saw Jake, with all the tubes sticking out of him, it was overwhelming. But the nurses were pretty good at explaining everything and the doctors were amazing. They would take as much time as we needed to explain what was going on, whether it was a procedure, a result, etc.

The best word: In short, it was amazing — getting through the process and having two amazing kids. My pregnancies were different because I had to do IVF with a donor egg and both kids were delivered C-section. I was also on bed rest with Jorja for 6 weeks, 4 of which were in the hospital. I feel so blessed and would do it again. I just wish I was a little younger when I did it.

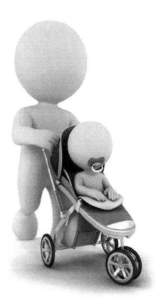

My advice to Type 1 diabetics: Do lots of research and prepare for the unknown. You might have a very normal pregnancy. But in case you don't, be prepared. I started on an insulin pump a year before we tried to get pregnant and I met with all the doctors and made my decisions on who I wanted to work with before we even started

~ Shelby W., Type 1 diabetes for over 20 years

∽

"A baby is an inestimable blessing and bother."
~ *Mark Twain, American author and humorist*

∽

> *When I was considering having a child my biggest concern was that my child would suffer the same fate as me and be forced to deal with diabetes. I lamented over the guilt I would feel if I passed this disease on to my child. I did not want to see my child face a low blood glucose in the middle of the night, or any of the social challenges that I have and still face.*
>
> *I was also in fear of having a low blood glucose episode myself. When a child is young, they are 100% dependent upon you. The thought of me not able to care for myself at a time when I was supposed to be caring for my child was very scary! In the end, I would not give Hannah back under any circumstances, but at this stage in my life, divorced and 40, I don't think I would consider having another child.*
>
> Matt B., Type 1 diabetes 28 years

I found a wonderful post on the blog, www.SixUntilMe.com from Jessica Hickok.

I am Type 1 diabetic and 31 years old. When I was 22, my husband and I had been married two years when we decided it was time to fulfill our dreams and have a baby. And the biggest piece of advice I can give to everyone who has seen the movie Steel Magnolias it is important to remember that life does not always imitate art.

We did the planning and really worked hard on keeping my blood sugars regulated. We spoke to my doctor, and with an HbA1c of 6.8%, we were given the green light to have a baby. <insert cheesy, romantic interlude here>.

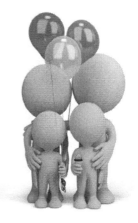

However, when I found out that I was pregnant with my first child, I was both elated and scared at the same time. I knew it was coming, but I immediately thought. "What if something goes wrong?" When other PWDs

(Persons with Diabetes) ask me about my child-birth experiences, I feel compelled to share my story and the following advice of what you can expect, or should consider:

1. Do not let diabetes steal your thunder

    Be happy for yourself. You're having a baby! Just because you have a chronic condition does not mean you cannot enjoy the pregnancy and anticipation of motherhood. Nor can you let your dreams be ruled by fear or guilt over your disease. So you have to work a little harder at staying in a healthy glucose range — big deal! You're going to do that anyway.

2. Be comfortable with your doctor

    Being diabetic automatically puts you in a high-risk category. However, that doesn't mean that you should lose sight of your basic rights as a patient. Find a doctor who is comfortable with your disease and is willing to work with your diabetes doctor or endocrinologist.

3. Expect that your baby might be big

    High sugars can spill over into the placenta feeding the baby and causing a large birth weight. Both of my boys were born approximately three weeks early and the first one weighed 9lbs. 12oz. My second was 10lbs. 14oz. No, I am not looking for a prize, but I do point that out just to prove that all of my complaining during pregnancy was justified.

4. You may have to have a cesarean section delivery

    C-sections aren't bad, they just sound scary. Yes, it will take you time to recover, but just think, with your tightly controlled blood sugars that you had during pregnancy, your recovery time should go relatively quick. I had both of my babies delivered by c-section and I wouldn't trade it for the world. I did tell you that they were big babies, right?

5. Expect your sugar readings to roller coaster after having the baby

    While my hormones were bouncing around back into place the few weeks after having the baby, it caused my sugar readings to bounce along with them.

6. Diabetics have healthy babies all the time

    Today, my first child is eight-years-old and my second is five-years-old. They are bright, healthy and so far, diabetes free. (Knock on wood.) And the good news is that my story didn't turn out at all like the one in Steel Magnolias.

    I was lucky to have my insulin pump while I was pregnant. And because there have been so many advances in diabetes technology (enter CGMS!), It has only become better and easier for diabetics to have children.

    The moment I held my precious newborn, my fears washed away. For those amazing first moments of holding my new baby, I was not diabetic. I was a mother.

Disclosure from Jessica: Please keep in mind that this post is written purely based on my opinion and my personal experiences with pregnancy and childbirth. I am not by any means a medical doctor. Nor do I share my story as medical advice. Please talk to your doctor about your plans to have children.

Jessica H., Type 1 diabetes for over 20 years

> *I was very lucky as a type 1 diabetic since childhood — to have had a healthy baby in 1973! Back then, there were no specialists. It was a conscious choice. The most important thing was that I gave birth naturally. I did not have to have a C-section. This was unheard of back then. And I did not have to spend any time in the hospital during my pregnancy. Also unheard of back then.*
>
> *So, my suggestion to any diabetic contemplating pregnancy — go for it!*
>
> Liz D., Type 1 diabetes for over 50 years

"If one feels the need of something grand,
something infinite,
something that makes one feel aware of God,
one need not go far to find it.

I think that I see something deeper,
more infinite, more eternal than the ocean
in the expression of the eyes of a little baby,
when it wakes in the morning and coos or laughs
because it sees the sun shining on its cradle."

~ Vincent Van Gogh, Dutchpost-impressionist painter

**A QUICK REVIEW OF KEY TOPICS:
HAVING BABIES OR NOT**

- Take time to consider your decision, the support around you and your access to knowledgeable medical systems.
- While babies of diabetics are often large, they can be delivered healthy and happy
- Prior and during pregnancy, you will need to very carefully monitor your blood glucose. Be prepared to work hard to deliver a healthy baby.

6.2 ~ Spouses, Partners, Families and Friends

"In every conceivable manner, the family is
link to our past, bridge to our future."
~*Alex Haley, American novelist*

KEY TOPICS

- When a family member is diagnosed with diabetes dynamics and relationships will be affected.
- There are issues at every age in living with diabetes
- There are resources available.

A Diabetic Child in the Family

I had just turned 11 when we learned I was diabetic. While it sometimes feels like just yesterday, I remember the terror I felt and the terror and guilt my mother felt. She cried a lot. I worried that my sister would get angry at me for getting so much attention. My dad spent a lot of time trying to busy himself with fundraising for a diabetes cure and charting my urine tests. It was a very difficult time for my family, and we were no different than any other family receiving the news that one of their children has diabetes.

Having a child with diabetes changes the dynamics of a family, whether you like it or not. If there are siblings, it's the perfect set up for jealousy (of the extra time spent with the sick child), anger, fear (the non-diabetic child might be afraid of catching the disease), sadness... the possibilities are endless. But you can be sure there will be some reaction among siblings.

What about the parents? How do they feel—about themselves, their sick child and their other children or other families not dealing with diabetes? Some parents feel guilt (they must have carried the wrong genes or done something to allow their child develop diabetes), some blame each other, some are terribly frightened, many deny it (maybe it will just go away)… again, so many possibilities.

The effects are felt beyond the immediate family, to the grandparents, cousins, and friends. Having a child with diabetes profoundly changes interactions, reactions, and communications. I can't even begin to address this issue. There are books available, as well as therapists, support groups, and diabetes associations to help.

What I can say is this: When a child is diagnosed with diabetes, it has a huge impact on everyone in that child's world. The child knows that, feels that, and has emotions tied up in all those dynamics. You, your child, and your family will most likely have to interact with the medical system for the rest of his or her life.

Be aware that a child with diabetes can also be a scary thing for friends. When I was in middle school and my blood glucose was low, I had to go to the nurse's office for juice. My best friend was assigned to take me there. We would giggle about how this was a great excuse to get out of class. I found out 30 years later that she was actually terrified that something would happen to me on the walk or that she might possibly catch the disease, too! How frightening that must be for children who don't fully understand much about the disease.

A Young Adult with Diabetes

In my teen years and throughout college, I just wanted to blend in, fit in, be regular. In retrospect, I did that fairly well, and I survived. But it was hard! I didn't always eat right, I didn't always take my medications regularly, and I often tried to ignore that fact that I had diabetes. So I had erratic blood glucose levels, and I may have done some damage to my body along the way.

What can we learn from this? Being a young person with diabetes is so very challenging. Allow for excursions from good diabetes care, but realize that taking care of ourselves will make us feel better and allow us to be "regular." After all, as a teenager, all we want is to be normal, just like everyone else. We want to fit in with our friends and not be bothered with all the details of everyday life with diabetes.

> *When we were teenagers, my friend Matt was diagnosed with Type 1 diabetes at age 14. We would go on surf trips, weekends to the river, etc., and he would "get low." We all would think that he was immature for not taking care of his diabetes. It would scare the c**p out of us and it would make the trips very stressful.*
>
> *But several years later, at the age of 22, I was diagnosed with Type 1 diabetes! And I now realize how difficult it is to manage diabetes. The tighter our control and the better we try to manage blood glucose fluctuations, the higher probability for low blood glucose episodes. Being a friend of a diabetic before I was diagnosed and being on both sides of the curtain, it is very easy to understand how people without the disease don't comprehend what people with diabetes go through on a day to day basis.*
>
> *It's not like we can just take our medication and be normal. It's "game on," all day long, every day. I don't think people without it really truly understand how difficult it really is. (Sorry, Matt, for all those years that your friends thought you didn't know how to take control of your diabetes.)*
>
> Justin M., Type 1 diabetes for 15 years

When I got to the age of dating and serious relationships, my mother told me she was frightened that no one would want to go out with me. She then advised me not to tell any guy about my diabetes until he was "hooked" on me and a relationship. There was one guy who stayed away from me when I told him I had diabetes. His father was a diabetic and he just didn't want to deal with a girlfriend with diabetes. I could totally understood his concerns.

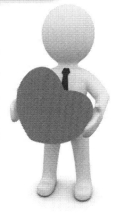

When I met my current husband, I told him on our first date, but that wasn't my plan.

We were having lunch at a charming German delicatessen. After we ate our sandwiches, he kept offering me bites of chocolate-covered marzipan. I took one bite, then another. Then I finally said, "I'm sorry but no more, I have diabetes."

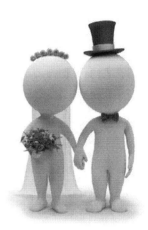

He looked quite stunned and then horrified with the thought that he was feeding me food that could hurt me. I settled him down by explaining that I was really ok with the two bites and knew what I was doing. As it turned out, his mother was a Type 1 diabetic, which then put me on high alert that he might run away.

He didn't run away! But despite over fifteen years together and all his reassurances that he won't leave because of my diabetes, I must say I still harbor that fear in the back of my mind to this day.

Spouses and Partners

He didn't run away, but he did something that seemed most unusual to me at the time. He became involved in understanding my medical program and was always concerned that I had all that I needed. Then, when we started to discuss marriage, he sought a consultation with an endocrinologist (not mine) to discuss his concerns and what he could expect, in the long run, if he married a Type 1 diabetic. When I found out that he did that, I was furious. He didn't first discuss it with me and he didn't speak to a doctor who was familiar with my conditions and how well I managed. Over time, I realized that he was just trying to be fully prepared so he could make an informed decision before he made a 100% commitment.

He certainly is committed 100%. He often participates in my doctors' appointments and consults with me on medication changes and health choices. He charts my data, doing regression analysis and statistics on my results (and proudly boasts results to those who will listen).

I know I can rely on him and he will not walk away if the going gets tough. For that, I am immensely grateful and fortunate.

Not every partner will do that or do all that you need, and it doesn't mean you are loved or cared for any less.

Whomever you choose (or have chosen) for a partner comes with pluses and minuses. But you must, as a diabetic, do what is necessary to ensure the level of support you need, on a daily basis as well as during emergencies that may pop up.

Being married to Type One Diabetic

My wife is a Type 1 diabetic. We've been together for 27 years — married for 25. So in many ways, I feel that I'm as connected to the disease as she is.

Of course, I'm not. I don't have the constant requirement to test my blood sugar, experience the roller coaster effects of high and low blood sugars, night sweats, the mood shifts and the unending attachment to the myriad of equipment that goes along with having Type 1 diabetes.

But I'm constantly aware of it all. Diabetes is the third person in our relationship — a person who is incredibly demanding and doesn't respect our schedule, our social life or our commitments.

My wife's insulin pump also plays a distinct role in our lives. It has a personality all of its own. It has an annoying tendency to go off at the most inopportune times. Like a child, it needs to be attended to when it needs to be attended to — no matter what it is you're doing at the moment.

In a weird way, I miss the good, old days when my wife tested her blood, whipped out her needle, measured the insulin and gave herself a shot. Like so much in our modern world, life has gotten more complicated as medical science has found new ways to deal with the disease.

Diabetes is emotionally draining — much more so for my wife than for me. But it is there — it's always there. And we both wish it would just go away.

Michael R., Type 1 diabetic for 30 years

How to Communicate

Here's my best advice: Learn to communicate!

I've learned a lot from Nonviolent Communication
(NVC or Compassionate Communication,
developed by Marshall Rosenberg in the 1960s):*

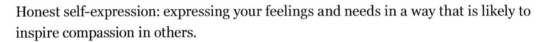

> Self-empathy: caring awareness of your
> own inner feelings and needs.

> Empathy: listening to another with
> caring compassion.

> Honest self-expression: expressing your feelings and needs in a way that is likely to
> inspire compassion in others.

With your spouse, partner, and any others (even your doctors), it is important to understand
what your own needs are, listen with compassion to the other's feelings and needs, and learn
to express yourself in ways that will get your needs met.

The subject is more than I can cover here. But my suggestion is that you learn to communicate
with kindness to those close to you and with those you interact. Understand, with kindness
and compassion, the needs and feelings of your partner, family, and friends.

When you are living with diabetes, it helps to remember:**

> You are responsible for meeting your own needs.

> People want to be heard and understood.

> The most meaningful connection is at the level of our humanness (not our diabetes)...
> what's alive in our feelings and our needs.

> When our needs and feelings are seen empathically, it stimulates natural compassion.

 * *Nonviolent Communication: A Language of Life by Marshall B. Rosenberg*
 ***Loving What Is: Four Questions that can Change Your Life by Byron Katie and Stephen Mitchell*

Reach out to Resources

You are not alone. Thousands of families are going through the same experience. For additional support, check out any local diabetes support group or diabetes center, certified diabetes educators (often on staff in your endocrinologist's office), American Diabetes Association, JDRF, Children with Diabetes website, Six Until Me blog. There are so many resources. I've listed several online sites at the back of the book. All you have to do is reach out and help will be there.

> *Love my pump and most especially love my Dexcom...of course, I get along well with my husband too! J*
>
> Mary Jo, Type 1 diabetes for 48 years

"If your husband has difficulty getting to sleep,
the words, 'we need to talk about our relationship' may help"
~ Rita Rudner, American comedian, dancer and writer

A QUICK REVIEW OF KEY TOPICS:
SPOUSES, PARTNERS, AND FAMILIES

- When a family member is diagnosed with diabetes, all the dynamics and relationships will be affected.
- There are specific issues with living with diabetes at every age (childhood, teen years, young adult, marriage and career building years, parenthood and grandparenthood).
- There are resources available to help at every stage of living with diabetes.

PART 7: COPING TOOLBOX

7.1   Anger, Fear, Gratitude and More

7.2   How to Talk to a Diabetic

7.3   A Place to Vent

7.4   Laughter is the Best Medicine

     ✧ Health benefits of a smile a day

     ✧ Fun with quotes

     ✧ Fun with Dr. Seuss-style

     ✧ Fun with cartoons

     ✧ Fun with jokes

7.5   Giving Back

Do you recognize these emotions? How many of them did you have today?

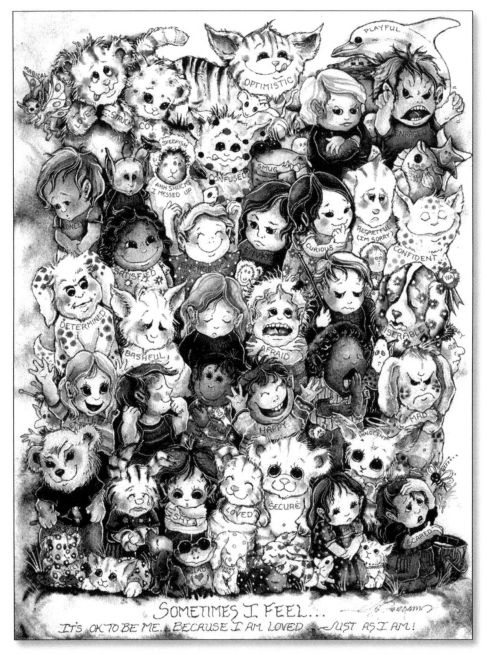

Permission to reprint, with much appreciation to Jody Bergsma, Bergsma Gallery, Bellingham, WA

7.1 ~ Anger, Fear, Gratitude and More

"When angry count to four.
When very angry, swear."
~ Mark Twain, American author and humorist

UNDERSTATEMENT: Type 1 Diabetes is a very challenging and devastating disease. With improved medications and technology, more and more Type 1 diabetics are living longer.

It is a 24/7 disease. It requires constant self-management and self-monitoring. One Type 1 diabetic estimated that she spent 456 hours /year, just in routine tasks and awareness of her blood glucose and insulin needs. That is almost nine hours EVERY WEEK to live with this disease and that estimate is CONSERVATIVE! Imagine what you could do with any extra 9-10 hours very week? All that "self-aware" time can be very tiresome and frustrating. And yet, we go on and we live our lives. Listen to some words from people who live with this disease.

> *This is a pretty awesome attitude from my little one! I picked her up from school yesterday and her class had been celebrating a classmate's birthday with cupcakes for everyone. The entire class ate them immediately but she had to take hers home so I could give her insulin.*
>
> *As we were driving home she tells the story and I'm feeling a bit sad for her so I asked how she felt. "Oh no, it's OK...they don't get to have a cupcake later like I do." She is wiser than her six years.*
>
> Anna R., Age 6, Type 1 diabetes for 3 years

A type-1 diabetic (T1D) since age nine, doctors have been ever present in my life for 40+ years now. I was in my early twenties when I first realized that doctors are not super-human; they're just smart people who managed to graduate medical school and then complete a subsequent hospital internship. Some are compassionate, some not, but few are diabetic and none can fully appreciate your unique life experience. The realization was transformative. I fired my endocrinologist, the one who regularly made me cry because I didn't conform to her textbook expectations, and instead sought out team members rather than task masters.

No one will ever care more about your health than you do. T1D is serious business and it's folly to suggest otherwise. Having good doctors is fundamentally important, but it's equally important to acknowledge the truth that you must be an active partner — your input matters! Surround yourself with a team of competent professionals whose counsel you value, but to thine own self be true. Pay attention to how your own unique body responds to treatments and feed your observations back to the team. If they ignore your inputs, find a new team.

Diabetes has thrown me many curve balls. Reflecting on those years, I realize what amazing strength I truly have.

There is a huge psychological element to diabetes. This disease is so consuming daily and long-term. Because I'm making calculations for endless variables, perfection doesn't exist.

Sharon, Type 1 diabetes for 40+ years

When I was diagnosed T1 in the 1970s there were few means for managing diabetes; I did urine testing, which I knew was fruitless even as a lay teenager. Diabetes management was based on strict regimens. Period. When blood testing became available this didn't change much. Diabetes experts seemed disconnected from their customers — people like me.

Twelve years later (most spent in denial, no surprise), I asked my doctor if there would ever be better way for people to live with diabetes. He smiled and said I shouldn't get my hopes up as a cure would not happen in my lifetime. He told me I could manage better with the help of a psychiatrist! The best thing I've ever done is to disregard this advice and move on.

Shortly thereafter I got an insulin pump. When continuous monitoring became available, I immediately got it. I've used the invaluable help of peers to leverage these tools and discover amazing things about diabetes. Running for a couple of hours without having to eat or having sugars go below/above normal the whole time has been called impossible, but we found a way!

My peers continue to be my most trusted, reliable, coveted sources of knowledge, and the sacred keys to my universe.

Jessica C., T1 diabetes for 33 years

> *Back in the early 1970s, when diabetes wasn't as well-known as it is now, a friend and I went to dinner. She, too, was a Type 1 diabetic. I mentioned that I hated going into the stall in the ladies room to take my dinner injection. She agreed and decided that we should liberate ourselves and just go into the ladies room near the sinks and take our injections.*
>
> *The time came.... and as we prepared to take our injections, a woman came out of one of the stalls, glared at us, and ran out. We continued with our injections and just at the point we each had a needle in our arm, the restaurant manager came into the ladies room. He asked us if we needed any help, to which my friend replied, no, actually, we are quite good at this.*
>
> *This was my very first coming out of the closet liberated moment.*
>
> Mary Jo, T1 diabetes for 48 years

Exercise helps!

I was just about to go to print on this book when I hadn't mentioned anything about exercise, a very critical part of controlling blood glucose and managing diabetes and coping with emotions. How could I forget? After graduate school, I started my own aerobics business, after work hours, for working professionals like myself. When I moved to the west coast, I continued to teach low-impact aerobics and yoga. It was fun to teach my classes and it guaranteed that I would get my exercise.

I continue to exercise almost daily. I don't always feel like it, I don't always want to, but I do. You have to figure out what works best for you and how to fit it in your lifestyle. Be sure to discuss your exercise goals and regimen with your healthcare providers. You will feel better with a little bit of workout. Here are just some examples, to get you motivated.

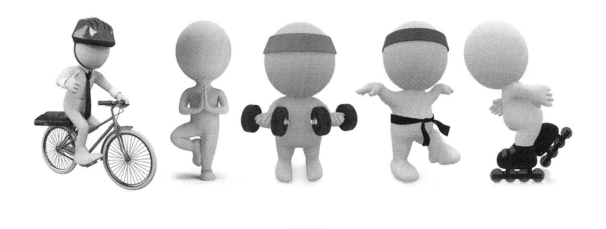

"You, yourself, as much as anybody in the entire universe,
deserve your love and affection."

~ Buddha, a sage from ancient Shakya, on whose teachings Buddhism was founded

When you feel it is getting to be "a bit too much," reach out! Talk with friends, support groups, your doctor. Maybe you can take a "diabetes time out" for a few hours.

This section is mostly about how we all cope, on a daily and even hourly basis with a disease that lives with us 24/7. It is so easy to get caught up in its urgency. But sometimes, you just have to step back and give yourself a pat on the back for a very difficult job very well done!

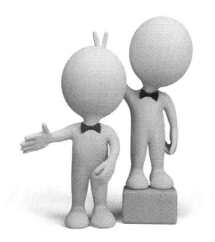

∽

"I wish I could show you, when you are lonely or in darkness,
the astonishing light of your own being."

~ Hafiz, 14th century Persian mystic and poet

∽

7.2 ~ How to Talk to a Diabetic

"The single biggest problem in communication
is the illusion that it has taken place."

~ *George Bernard Shaw, Irish playwright and economist*

What to Say: Do's and Don'ts

People often say unfortunate things. They will tell you about all their relatives or acquaintances who had diabetes and who had amputations, went blind, or died from kidney failure. They will tell you this while you are eating. Sometimes, they will become the "food police," and try to monitor what you are eating by telling you what you should or should not eat or drink. They offer suggestions on how to manage your health. And depending on how you are feeling on any given day, you might just brush off their comments with a smile or get really upset at their insensitivities and rude assumptions.

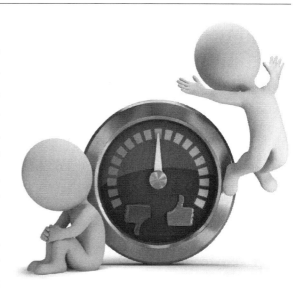

Here are some comments we sometimes hear, through our diabetic ears:

➢ You have diabetes? I know how you feel. I'm allergic to peanut butter!

➢ You have diabetes?! Oh my gosh, I couldn't take shots!! I would just kill myself!!

➢ You play sports?! But I thought you were diabetic!

➢ When ordering a drink at a restaurant: Diet coke?! You don't need to be on a diet!

➢ Do you have the bad kind of diabetes?

➢ Is that an iPod? (No it's not an iPod, it's my insulin pump.)

➢ Does your insulin pump have games on it?

- ➢ Is that heroin in your pump?
- ➢ Knew a girl who had type 1 diabetes, she died when she was 30.
- ➢ You can't eat that!
- ➢ You got diabetes from eating too many sweets.
- ➢ Can you test my blood sugar with your pricky finger thingy?!
- ➢ My best friend's neighbor's uncle's boss's wife had diabetes, and she cured it through diet and exercise. You should try it.
- ➢ Awww, you have diabetes? My cat has diabetes too! (This one is my favorite!)
- ➢ Well, at least you don't have cancer.

The list goes on. Sometimes, these comments come from ignorance, sometimes from fear. Sometimes they make me laugh, sometimes they make me cringe, and sometimes they just hurt.

Dr. Bill Polonsky, founder of the Behavioral Diabetes Institute in San Diego, CA, has developed a Diabetes Etiquette Card for people who don't have diabetes. It's a precious fold-out card that you can hand out to friends and coworkers, and even medical professionals.

Topics include the following Do's and Don'ts:
- ➢ Don't offer unsolicited advice about my eating.
- ➢ Do realize and appreciate that diabetes is hard work.
- ➢ Don't tell me horror stories about your grandmother or others.
- ➢ Do offer to join me in making healthy lifestyle changes.
- ➢ Don't look so horrified when I check my blood glucose or give myself an injection.
- ➢ Do ask how you might be helpful.
- ➢ Don't offer thoughtless reassurances.
- ➢ Do be supportive of my efforts for self-care.
- ➢ Don't peek at or comment on my blood glucose numbers.
- ➢ Do offer your love and encouragement.

You can order cards for $1 from BDI or download a PDF from their website: www.behavioraldiabetesinstitute.org.

~

"When ignorance gets started, it knows no bounds."

~ *Will Rogers, American cowboy, humorist, social commentator and actor*

~

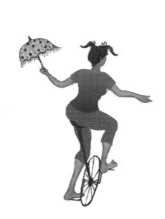

7.3 ~ A Place to Vent

"Life is not always fair.
Sometimes you get a splinter even sliding down a rainbow."

~ *Terri Guillemets, American quotation anthologist*

 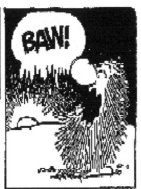 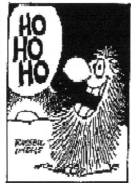 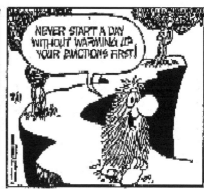

We have all these thoughts that run around in our heads, all the time. Everyone does.

But for a diabetic, we have a whole extra layer of concerns and feelings, and they are all valid and real.

Sometimes it's good to write them down, all of them. The positive thoughts like the ones where we feel gratitude and faith. The negative ones are the ones that express our anger, frustration, weariness, sadness, and fear.

And more.

Here's my extended list:

1. Lost time: Sometimes I feel so dang tired that I can't do anything. There is also the time lost waiting for low blood sugars to come up, or high blood sugars to come down.

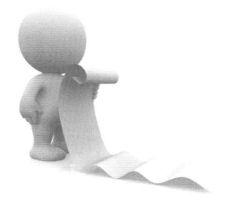

2. Interruptions: I hate when I have to stop what I'm doing to deal with a diabetes related issue.

3. Messing up plans: Life is busy. When I have a day where I can go play, only to have my blood sugar not cooperate, it really frustrates me.

4. Cost: Living well with diabetes is expensive.

5. Unpredictability: Even when I do things exactly the same from day to day, diabetes doesn't respond the same.

6. Seeing people I care about hurting, physically and/or mentally emotionally.

7. Having to be so damn prepared for everything — my mind is always calculating "what if" scenarios. Always.

8. Food: Diabetes has made food become something different than just food.

9. Counting, figuring, factoring: I can't remember three digit numbers (like a parking space) because my head is overflowing with random diabetes related numbers.

10. When you realize you'd never survive stranded on a deserted island.

11. Stuff that hurts: Pokes, blood, stuff sticking into me, wires and cables hanging off me. So unnatural.

12. Always waiting for the next shoe to drop.

13. I'm required to expect the unexpected at all times. This means carrying insulin, pump supplies, glucose, meter, etc. each time I leave my house. I've paid the price for not being prepared.

14. When you get a package in the mail and get excited, then realize it's just diabetes supplies.

15. The consequences of not being perfect are immediate and long-term. Shocker: I'm not perfect.

16. I just get tired of diabetes.

17. When your insulin pump tubing gets caught on EVERYTHING! Rings, belts, doorknobs, steering wheels.

18. I want to go on a vacation and leave my diabetes at home.

19. People asking me why my blood sugar is high or low at a particular time.

20. People questioning what I should or shouldn't be eating.

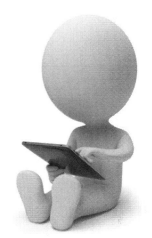

And I'm sure you can add to the list. And please do! As thoughts and feelings come to mind, please post them at my blog: www.TheSavvyDiabetic.com and I'll try to include them in our next printing.

> *I feel alone, scared when I'm alone, and I get very tired of dealing with it every day. Sometimes I feel like it would be nice just to have a weekend off every few months. That would be great. To cope, I hang with other diabetics. I have to stay positive and motivated.*
>
> *I know diabetes has made me a better person, a better listener, a better husband, a better father, and a healthier person.*
>
> *I know this sounds weird but I feel life with diabetes has been a much more fulfilling life. I have learned so much more and have become a happier person.*
>
> Justin M., Type 1 diabetes, 15+ years

7.4 ~ Laughter is the Best Medicine

I will not play tug o' war.
I'd rather play hug o' war.
Where everyone hugs instead of tugs,
Where everyone giggles and rolls on the rug,
Where everyone kisses, and everyone grins,
and everyone cuddles, and everyone wins.

~ Shel Silverstein, American poet, singer-song-writer, cartoonist, author

I have been blessed with a sense of humor, I think. I seem to have the ability to find a smile, in the midst of some of the harsher times in life. And I deeply feel that humor, smiling, laughter, and giggles are our savior during great stress.

SMILE: n. or v.: [smīl] a facial expression formed by flexing the muscles near both ends of the mouth and by flexing muscles throughout the mouth. Some smiles include contraction of the muscles at the corner of the eyes. Among humans, it is an expression denoting pleasure, sociability, happiness, or amusement.

HUMOR: n. [hyü-mər]

1. *The quality that makes something laughable or amusing; funniness.*
2. *That which is intended to induce laughter or amusement.*

LAUGHTER: n. [laf-tər] to show emotion with a chuckle or explosive vocal sound.

GIGGLE: n. or v. [gi-gəl] to laugh with repeated short catches of the breath.

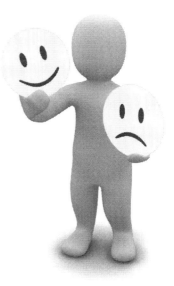

There is a lot written in the medical literature about the healing power of laughter. One website states that laughter is good for your health:

Laughter relaxes the whole body. A good, hearty laugh relieves physical tension and stress, leaving your muscles relaxed for up to 45 minutes after.

Laughter boosts the immune system. Laughter decreases stress hormones and increases immune cells and infection-fighting antibodies, thus improving your resistance to disease.

Laughter triggers the release of endorphins, the body's natural feel-good chemicals. Endorphins promote an overall sense of well-being and can even temporarily relieve pain.

Laughter protects the heart. Laughter improves the function of blood vessels and increases blood flow, which can help protect you against a heart attack and other cardiovascular problems.

Norman Cousins, who served as Adjunct Professor of Medical Humanities for the School of Medicine at the University of California, Los Angeles, long believed that laughter is the key to human being's success in fighting illness. His book, Anatomy of an Illness, is must reading in our struggles to cope with and survive with diabetes.

And veteran comedian, Craig Shoemaker, a self-described "modern day Renaissance man," has been making audiences laugh since attending Temple University in Philadelphia, PA, his hometown. Craig has had several successful solo TV stand-up specials, co-starred in numerous films, hosted popular network TV shows, written two beloved children's books and performed for four U.S. Presidents. 'Dr. Shoe' has a doctorate degree from Cal U of PA, is an ordained minister, and has one Best Comedian awards many times over. In 2003, he launched a website called: Laughter Heals (www.LaughterHeals.org), whose goal is to promote healing through laughter, as a tribute to his best friend, Mike Polin, who lost his struggle with cancer.

Play with a little diabetes-related humor and see if it touches your funny bone or giggle switch.

Fun with quotes

Start every day off with a smile and get it over with.

W. C. Fields

The more I live, the more I think that humor is the saving sense.

Jacob August Riis

One doesn't have a sense of humor. It has you.

Larry Gelbart

Humor can alter any situation and help us cope at the very instant we are laughing.

Allen Klein

A well-developed sense of humor is the pole that adds balance to your steps
as you walk the tightrope of life.

William Arthur Ward

When humor goes, there goes civilization.

Erma Bombeck

Comedy is simply a funny way of being serious.

Peter Ustinov

A day without sunshine is like, you know, night.

Steve Martin

Ever notice how 'What the hell' is always the right answer?

Marilyn Monroe

Be careful about reading health books. You may die of a misprint.

Mark Twain

I generally avoid temptation unless I can't resist it.

Mae West

I refuse to answer that question on the grounds that I don't know the answer.

Douglas Adams

Fun with Dr. Seuss*

Lancets! Test strips! Testing now! I can, you can, we know how.
Look! See! Blood drops, one and two and three.

Why won't this meter beep for me?
Numbers now. Number's high! 182 — my, oh my!

Out with the insulin, out with the needle
Out with the afternoon snack-n-feedle.

Corrections, ouch. Corrections ooch.
Injections 10x/day hurt my hooch.

Up, up, up and down the stairs — Now I'm taking stairs in pairs.
Down with the glucose readings! Down, down, down!

I'll have the best numbers in any town.
Funny, now I cannot think... Think what I thunk and my heart begins to sink.

Oops! Up with the sugar level — up, up, up!
Glucose tablets, gummi drops, and orange juice in a big, BIG cup.

But, see! High again, that's where I am. Above 150, gosh darn damn.
And on it goes throughout the day. Look, what fun! Come on and play.

But if we sweat, then we must eat. But not a treat! No, not a treat!
Round and round and round it goes, and where it stops could be my toes.

I'd like to keep mine. Yes, that's wise. I'll keep my nerves and feet and eyes.
I'd like to keep them all, mind you... So I'll do what I have to do.

But like it? No, no, no, I say!
I do not like the vials, the rules, the thinking, worrying all day.

I do not like it one little bit.
Still, I'm glad to LIVE with it.

Amy Tenderich, Founder and Editor of www.DiabetesMine.com

Fun with Cartoons

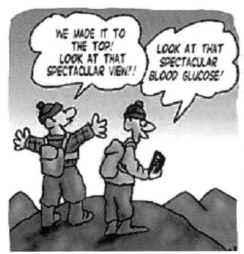

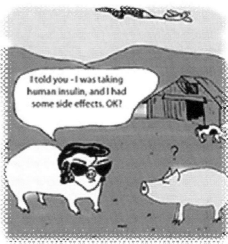

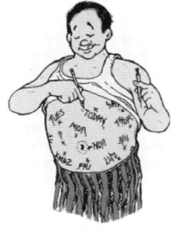

Because he knew the importance of daily injection site rotation, George went to extremes to avoid problems.

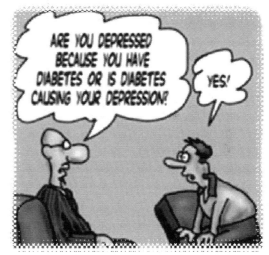

Fun with Jokes

Q: What does one meter say to another?
A: HI-LO

A Diabetic walks into a bakery as asks the guy behind the counter,
"Whaddya got that is safe for diabetics?"
The Baker says, "Everything. As long as you don't put it in your mouth."

What city has the most diabetics per capita?
Needles, California.

I didn't find many jokes that made me laugh. If you come across some, please send them my way: www.TheSavvyDiabetic.com

7.5 ~ Giving Back

We make a living by what we get,
but we make a life by what we give.
~ Winston Churchill, British politician and prime minister

Ever since I was diagnosed, I have been involved with fundraising to find a cure. That's a lot of years of fundraising. My dad used to run the Rolls Royce raffle to fund diabetes research in the early 1970s. Each raffle cost $100, and the raffle was limited to 500 chances. Every business meeting my dad held started with him selling a Rolls Royce raffle ticket. Then he would conduct his business. He was just so committed to helping his little girl!

I have been carrying on the tradition for years, both in fundraising and outreach to other diabetics, both children and adults. It's bad enough to have to deal with this devastating and difficult disease. The least I can do is share my experiences, knowledge, and maybe raise awareness and money to find a cure.

Since 1995, I have captained a Walk team, called the Shooting Stars. The name came us in a team planning meeting in the days before I was pumping insulin, and I was just "shooting insulin" via syringe. I get tremendous support from family, friends, my medical team, and business associates and in the process, we all have a wonderful time.

"We must all hang together or most assuredly
we shall hang separately."
*~ Benjamin Franklin, American author, printer, political theorist, politician, postmaster,
scientist, musician, inventor, satirist, civic activist, statesman, and diplomat.*

Here are some photos of our team, over the past 18 years. A heartfelt thank you, Shooting Stars!

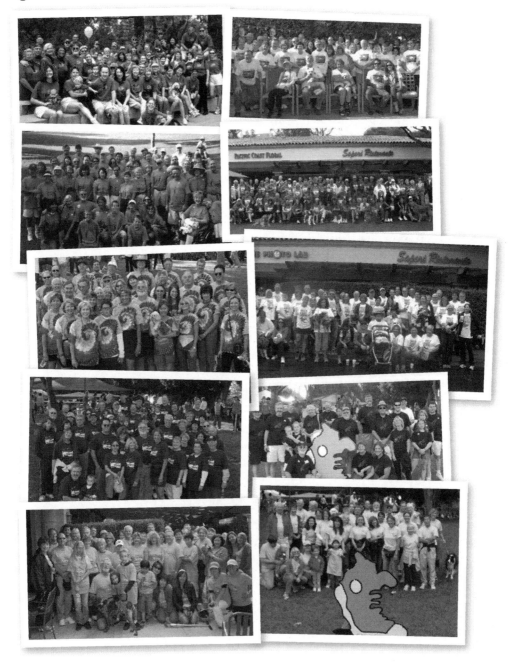

Part 8: Final Words

8.1   Top Ten List

8.2   What's Next?

8.3   Appreciations

8.4   In Remembrance

8.5   About the Author

8.1 ~ Top Ten List

This book is filled with lots of tips, tools, and techniques to guide you through this life journey with diabetes.

Do I do every on this list, always, consistently? No, of course not! Would it be wise if I did? Yes, of course! But I also have a life to live, a job to do, a family to interact with, dogs to play with. And I also sometimes just get plain tired of paying so much attention to my health and my diabetes. There, I said it and it's the truth.

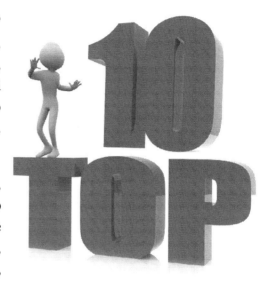

Below you will find the Top Ten List of tips, tools, and techniques from this book. If you only do three or four of them, you are still ahead of the game. If possible, choose from the top of the list, the more important items. If you do all ten items, drop me an email so I can cheer you on!

1. Buy and wear a medical ID tag which specifies your type of diabetes and any other important conditions, allergies or contact information.

2. Make a list of all your medications, allergies, emergency contacts and doctors.

3. Store your lists on a flash drive or carry a hard copy with you.

4. Update your lists every quarter or when something changes significantly.

5. Choose those people who can serve as advocates for you.

6. Train your advocates on what you need them to know and understand about managing your diabetes.

7. Make a list of items you would need if you were going to be hospitalized.

8. Keep a stash of quick sugar and snacks with you, at your office desk and in your car.

9. Give yourself and your significant others appreciation as often as possible.

10. Choose to laugh or giggle or smile once a day.

Remember, you can be prepared by keeping your *The Savvy Diabetic: On The Go* workbook up-to-date and ready to go, available on www.TheSavvyDiabetic.com

❧

"When I see the Ten Most Wanted Lists,
I always have this thought:
If we'd made them feel wanted earlier,
they wouldn't be wanted now."
~ Eddie Cantor, American performer, comedian,
dancer, singer, actor, songwriter

❧

8.2 ~ What's Next?

I started to think about writing this book after several hospitalizations in a four year period. Up until then, I had studiously avoided hospitals, and had always been quite concerned. No, maybe terrified is the more accurate word, terrified, about being out of control in managing my diabetes and at the mercy of hospital personnel.

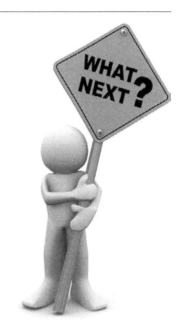

And then, on a dark and stormy night, it happened... an emergency, out of my control. And wow, did I learn!

What you have read in this book is a collection of suggestions, borne out of my experiences, as well as those of other diabetics. I hope you never have to be hospitalized. But, if you do, you are now armed with tips, tools and techniques to improve the experience, improve the outcome and put your mind at peace.

As I've been writing this, I find myself more and more drawn into diabetics' stories about coping and family. The essence of being successful with diabetes seems to be just darn luck and the ability to cope.

～

"Unless someone like you cares a whole awful lot,
nothing is going to get better. It's not."
~ Dr. Seuss, American writer, poet and cartoonist

～

8.3 ~ Appreciations

"Too much of a good thing can be wonderful!"
~ Mae West, American actress, singer, playwright and sex symbol

I received a lot of input and experiences, from diabetics, spouses, doctors, nurses, and friends.

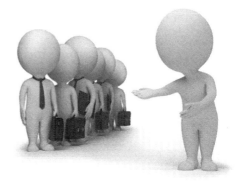

In particular, I owe my inspiration to GNO (Girls' Night Out), a group of amazing Type 1 diabetic women, all dynamos in their own lives and just the most supportive and kind collection of friends. I credit my MasterMind group, Lynn Smith, for getting me started, and Christy Jones, for holding my feet to the fire to complete this project as well as all the editing and formatting and brainstorming, and believing in me, a truly amazing friend, Donna Hayden for watching the kids while the adult diabetics talked, and Dr. Timothy Ryan, my spiritual guide.

I've gotten so much help, encouragement and advice along the way. More thanks to Marla Noel, who directed me to the Pen On Fire Speakers Series); and Barbara DeMarco-Barrett, host of Pen on Fire Speakers Series and an amazing editor and writing instructor, Tom Davis; Ken South; Mayor Robert Ming; Amy F. Ryan (author of Shot: Staying Alive with Diabetes); Dr. Mark Markowitz; Dr. Jonathan White, of Welcome to Type 1; Harrison Hughes, CureDiabetesBlog.com; Terri Brewster; Lois Levine; Monica Warthen, a fantastic proofreader; Jean Hobart and Jerry Von Talge; Tyler Reid; Jason Gallagher; insulin-pumpers.org; Linda Riley, Executive Director of JDRF, Orange County, CA; Lorraine Stiel; Gloring Loring; the late Janet Zorn; my late mom and dad, Audrey and Alfred, both of whom ached when I was diagnosed and would have gladly become diabetic to take it away from me; Dwight Sawin, my first boyfriend who showed me that it didn't matter that I had diabetes; Deborah Gould (my high school Frosted Flakes partner) and her brother, Dr. Eric Gould, who found me a wonderful surgeon at 7:00am; Alexis Stoniea, my constant cheerleader; and Cat Frecceri, ever enthusiastic and encouraging.

A special and heartfelt thank you to the most wonderful medical advisors and healthcare professionals, for their time and insight and enthusiasm... and amazing reviews! To the BEST of the BEST: Dr. Steven Edelman, Dr. Bill Polonsky, Dick Allen, Gloring Loring, Dr. Francine Kaufman, Dr. Daniel Einhorn, Robyn Nelson, Dr. Ping Wang, Dr. Athena Philis-Tsimikas, and John Walsh.

My technology gurus are the best! An enormous hug and thanks to Ray Sanford, Sanford Web Systems, always at the ready to help and guide me and save me from myself and Word; Ryan McCoy, Fewtr Technology, for the beautiful and creative web designs and book cover layout, over so many revisions; Joe Tranchida, MCS Computers who always keeps my computer up and running, even responding to urgent phone calls; Catherine Crahan; and Josh Yocam, a social media whiz at Oppenheimer.

And my very special heart goes out to all my GNO-ers: Sharon and John Roberson; Dale and Ted Rosenfeldt;, Karen Hill; Jessica Ching; Kim Williams; Casey Orr; Priscilla Faubel; Matt Besley; Sandra States; Susan Bohuslavizki; Justin Macklin; Marianne Plunkett; Linda and Michael Robertson; Suzie Won; and Bob & Diana Rourke and their sweet little Anna.

And I am eternally and forever grateful to my husband Richard who was by my side for every single trip to the hospital and helped me organize myself to be able to survive the system. He plotted my meter data, showed me trends, got up in the middle of the night to get me juice from the kitchen, and way too much to even describe. He is my shining knight, full of creativity and direction, always helpful and loving!

I must also mention Hey Buddy, my Westie, and Bon Bon, my Lhasa Apso, who kept me company and kept me amused during all the hours of my writing and also during all the hours of my many recoveries from surgery. (You may notice that Hey Buddy is holding his doctor squeak toy, which provides all of us with many hours of laughter.)

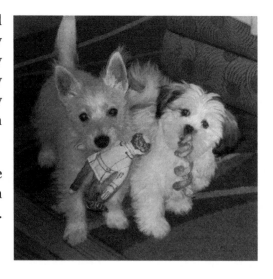

If I missed anything important that you have experienced and learned from, please share them with me and I'll include them in the next printing.

I truly hope this book is helpful to you and those around you. Please tell other diabetics and your medical team about this survival guide, so that they can better survive the system.

With the utmost humility and heartfelt appreciation, thank you for reading this book, using these tips, tools, and techniques, and sharing with others.

Joanne Laufer Milo
Corona del Mar, CA
Copyright 2013

8.4 ~ In Remembrance

My dear friend, Janet Zorn, who, at the age of 33, was taken far too soon
by the ravages of Type 1 diabetes complications.

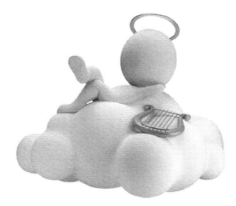

We met at the office of our ophthalmologist in New York City and became fast friends.

We shared our stories, our struggles with diabetes and most of all, our laughter.

Janet's laugh would light up her face and bring smiles to everyone around her.

Her sudden death after surgery for a diabetes complication was just so difficult.
It's been over 20 years and I still miss her.

Janet, I hope you are still bringing joy and love to all who are touched by you.

"There are no goodbyes for us.
Wherever you are, you will always be in our hearts."
~ *Mahatma Gandhi, Preeminent leader of Indian Nationalism*
and proponent of non-violent civil disobedience

8.5 ~ About the Author

"Draw your chair up close to the edge of the precipice
and I'll tell you a story."
~ *F. Scott Fitzgerald, American author of novels and short stories*

Joanne Laufer Milo was born and raised in the suburbs of New York City. She has a BA in psychology and mathematics from Union College in Schenectady, NY, along with an MBA in marketing from The Wharton School of the University of Pennsylvania in Philadelphia. She spent many years in marketing, particularly in new technologies (her favorite was in the field of artificial intelligence). After many years in the corporate world, she started an exercise, aerobics, and yoga business, figuring that making money while exercising would be a healthier way to live. She even had the fun privilege of working for Richard Simmons in his Anatomy Asylum Studios in Los Angeles.

Her great love of dogs started with her first two dogs, King Louis XIV, a white miniature poodle, and then later a precious toy poodle, Ginger. Joanne's passion for dogs lead to the formation of her website selling dog related art and gifts (www.3DogArt.com).

Joanne currently shares her life and love with Richard, her husband, whom she met when she placed a personal ad in the local newspaper, and their two joyful pups. The dogs are named Hey Buddy, a Westie (whose middle name is I'm Busy), and Bon Bon, the sweetest Lhasa Apso

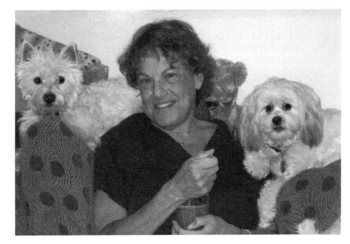

Joanne is blessed with loving friends and feels great joy and gratitude when she is able to share and help others in coping with this devastating disease. She has been volunteering with Juvenile Diabetes Foundation (JDRF) since its inception in the early 1970s in NYC and is now involved with the JDRF Tightrope T1D Outreach Committee, as well as Girls' (and now Guys') Night Out, a local support group for Type 1 diabetics and their significant others in Orange County, CA.

～

"And will you succeed? Yes, indeed, yes indeed!
Ninety-eight and three-quarters percent guaranteed!"

~ Dr. Seuss, American writer, poet and cartoonist

～

PART 9: APPENDIX

9.1   Resources and References

9.2   Glossary

9.3   Sample Medical Information Lists

♦ My sample lists

♦ MyMedicineList blank forms

♦ MedicAlert blank form and wallet card

9.4   Sample Hospital Diet Plans and Menus

9.5   TSA Information for Travelers, 2013

9.6   Foreign Language Translations

9.7   Conversion Charts

♦ Blood Glucose: mg/dl and mmol/L

♦ Centigrade and Fahrenheit

9.1 ~ Resources & References

"Today is your day! Your mountain is waiting.
So... get on your way."

~ Dr. Seuss, American writer, poet and cartoonist

Research and Fund Raising Organizations

American Diabetes Association

www.diabetes.org

Diabetes Hands Foundation

To connect, engage, and empower people touched by diabetes

www.diabeteshandsfoundation.org

Diabetes Research Institute Foundation

"The Best Hope for a Cure"

www.diabetesresearch.org

JDRF Improving Lives. Curing Type 1 Diabetes

(Formerly Juvenile Diabetes Research Foundation)

www.jdrf.org

Padre Foundation

Pediatric-Adolescent Diabetes Research Education Foundation

www.padrefoundation.org

Type 1 Diabetes TrialNet

An international network of researchers who are exploring ways to prevent, delay and reverse the progression of type 1 diabetes.

www.diabetestrialnet.org

Insulindependence

To reduce the burden of diabetes in the United States through physical activity and peer support, and to unite, expand, and support the active diabetes community.

www.insulindependence.org

Insulin for Life USA

Collects in-date and unneeded insulin, test strips as well as other diabetes supplies and ships them to developing countries
www.ifl-usa.org

Medical Supplies, Pumps and CGMS

Abbott Diabetes Care, makers of CGMS and blood glucose meters
www.abbottdiabetescare.com

Animas, makers of insulin pumps
www.animas.com

Asante Solutions, makers of the Snap insulin pump
www.SnapPump.com

Dexcom, maker of CGMS
www.dexcom.com

Insulet Omnipod, maker of tube-free insulin pumps
www.myomnipod.com

Medtronic, makers of insulin pumps and CGMS
www.medtronicdiabetes.com

Roche Diabetes Care, makers of blood glucose meters and insulin pump
www.accu-chek.com

Tandem, makers of the t:slim insulin pumps - www.tandemdiabetes.com

Technology and Website Resources

LiveScribe Smart Pens
www.livescribe.com

Calorie King, for calorie and carb counting
www.CalorieKing.com

Tidepool, applications that allow you to see ALL your data, via the "cloud", on smartphones
http://.tidepool.org

NightScout, open source DIY project that allows real time access to CGM to smart phones and smart watches
www.nightscout.info

Wearable Medical ID and Products

MedicAlert Foundation: Stores your medical information, contacts and doctors in their database, accessible via an 800 number. Also offers medical emblems and wallet card.
www.MedicAlert.org

Lauren's Hope: offers a large selection of fashion medical ID jewelry for men, women and children.
www.LaurensHope.com

RoadID: "It's Who I Am" sells durable, rugged, athletic, fashionable identification gear, including bands for your wrist, ankle, or shoe.
www.RoadID.com

Pump Wear: selling fun and kicky insulin pump cases and clothing
www.PumpWearInc.com

Myabetic: diabetes accessories for insulin pumps, diabetes supplies and CGMS.
www.mMyabetic.com

Frio: makes unique products for keeping insulin cool.
www.insulincoolingcase.com

Skidaddle: bags for carrying diabetes supplies.
www.skidaddlebags.com

SPIbelt: a "diabetic SPIbelt" to accommodate essential diabetes supplies.
www.spibelt.com

Bands4Life: arm, thigh and stomach bands to hold CGMS monitors and other diabetes supplies in place and secure, as well as Medical ID alert jewelry.
www.bands4life.net

Sticky Jewelry, functional and fashionable medical alert jewelry
www.StickyJ.com

Great Websites and Blogs

www.TheSavvyDiabetic.com: "A collection of tips, tools, and techniques to help you stay in control and balance, living with diabetes."

www.DiabetesMine.com: "A gold mine of straight talk and encouragement for people living with diabetes."

www.DiaTribe.us: "Research and product news for people with diabetes."

DiabetesCGMS Yahoo User Forum: "Email discussion list devoted to the topic of CGMS for diabetes."

www.TuDiabetes.com: "A social network for support, education, and sharing the steps taken every day to stay healthy while living with diabetes."

www.DiabetesDelicateBalance.blogspot.com: "To provide an outlet and support for people partnering in their loved one's fight to manage diabetes well."

www.discussdiabetes.com: "Connecting. Sharing. Learning..."

www.SixUntilMe.com: blog of a Type 1 diabetic who is also a freelance author. "Diabetes doesn't define me, but it helps explain me.

http://diabeteshealth.com: Investigate. Inform. Inspire."

www.curediabetesblog.com: "Inspiring Diabetics to Success in Life."

www.Childrenwithdiabetes.com: "The online community for kids, families, and adults with diabetes."

www.DiabetesDaily.com: "An online community for people with diabetes."

www.ScottsDiabetes.com: "My struggles, my successes, and everything in between."

http://asweetlife.org: by a couple who both have Type 1 diabetes

SweetlyVoiced.com

DSMA (Diabetes Social Media Advocacy): www.blogtalkradio.com/diabetessocmed

Diabetes Sisters at https://diabetessisters.org

9.2 ~ Glossary

Antibodies: Proteins made by the body to protect itself from "foreign" substances such as bacteria or viruses. People develop Type 1 diabetes when their bodies make antibodies that destroy the body's own insulin-making beta cells.

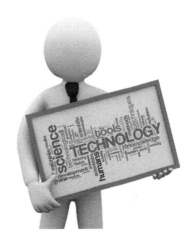

Autoimmune disease: A disorder of the body's immune system in which the immune system mistakenly attacks the body itself. Examples of these diseases include type 1 diabetes, hyperthyroidism caused by Graves' disease, and hypothyroidism caused by Hashimoto's disease.

Basal rate: The amount of insulin required to manage normal daily blood glucose fluctuations. Most people constantly produce insulin to manage the glucose fluctuations that occur during the day. In a person with diabetes, giving a constant low level amount of insulin via insulin pump mimics this normal phenomenon.

Beta cell: A type of cell in an area of the pancreas called the islets of Langerhans. Beta cells make and release insulin, which helps control the glucose level in the blood.

Blood glucose meter: A method of testing how much sugar is in your blood. Home blood-glucose monitoring involves pricking your finger with a lancing device, putting a drop of blood on a test strip and inserting the test strip into a blood-glucose-testing meter that displays your blood glucose level. Blood-sugar testing can also be done in the laboratory.

Bolus: an extra amount of insulin taken to cover an expected rise in blood glucose, often related to a meal or snack.

C-peptide: "Connecting peptide," a substance the pancreas releases into the bloodstream in equal amounts to insulin. A test of C-peptide levels shows how much insulin the body is making.

Carb Counting: a method of meal planning for people with diabetes based on counting the number of grams of carbohydrate in food.

Carbohydrate: One of the three main classes of foods and a source of energy. Carbohydrates are mainly sugars and starches that the body breaks down into glucose (a simple sugar that the body can use to feed its cells).

CDE (Certified Diabetes Educator): A health care professional that is certified by the American Association of Diabetes Educators (AADE) to teach people with diabetes how to manage their condition.

CT (CAT scan or Computed Axial Tomography): medical imaging procedure that utilizes computer-processed x-rays to produce tomographic images ("slices") of specific areas of the body.

Endocrinologist: A doctor who treats people with hormone problems.

Fats: Substances that help the body use some vitamins and keep the skin healthy. They are also the main way the body stores energy. In food, there are many types of fats — saturated, unsaturated, polyunsaturated, monounsaturated, and trans fats.

Flash drive (Jump drive, USB): data storage device, removable and rewritable, that includes flash memory with an integrated USB interface.

Gestational diabetes: A high blood sugar level that starts or is first recognized during pregnancy. Hormone changes during pregnancy affect the action of insulin, resulting in high blood sugar levels. Usually, blood sugar levels return to normal after childbirth. However, women who have had gestational diabetes are at increased risk of developing type 2 diabetes later in life. Gestational diabetes can increase complications during labor and delivery and increase the rates of fetal complications related to the increased size of the baby.

Glucose: A simple sugar found in the blood. It is the body's main source of energy; also known as "dextrose."

Glycemic Index: a ranking of carbohydrate-containing foods, based on the food's effect on blood glucose compared with a standard reference food.

Glycogen: the form of glucose found in the liver and muscles.

Hemoglobin A1c (HbA1c): This is an important blood test to determine how well you are managing your diabetes. Hemoglobin is a substance in red blood cells that carries oxygen to tissues. It can also attach to sugar in the blood, forming a substance called glycated hemoglobin or a Hemoglobin A1C. The test provides an average blood sugar measurement over a 6- to 12-week period and is used in conjunction with home glucose monitoring to make treatment adjustments. The ideal range for people with diabetes is generally less than 7%. This test can also be used to diagnose diabetes when the HbA1c level is equal to or greater than 6.5%.

Humalog: fast acting insulin analogue marketed by Eli Lilly and Company.

Human Insulin (insulin analog): an altered form of insulin, different from any occurring in nature, but still available to the human body for performing the same action as human insulin in terms of glycemic control. Through genetic engineering of the underlying DNA, the amino acid sequence of insulin can be changed to alter its ADME (absorption, distribution, metabolism, and excretion) characteristics. Officially, the U.S. Food and Drug Administration (FDA) refers to these as "insulin receptor ligands", although they are more commonly referred to as insulin analogs.

Hyperglycemia: High blood sugar. This condition is fairly common in people with diabetes. Many things can cause hyperglycemia. It occurs when the body does not have enough insulin or cannot use the insulin it does have.

Hypoglycemia: Low blood sugar. The condition often occurs in people with diabetes. Most cases occur when there is too much insulin and not enough glucose in your body.

Hormone: A chemical released in one organ or part of the body that travels through the blood to another area, where it helps to control certain bodily functions. For instance, insulin is a hormone made by the beta cells in the pancreas and when released, it triggers other cells to use glucose for energy.

Human Insulin: Bio-engineered insulin very similar to insulin made by the body. The DNA code for making human insulin is put into bacteria or yeast cells and the insulin made is purified and sold as human insulin.

Infusion Set: used with an insulin pump as part of intensive insulin therapy. The purpose of an infusion set is to deliver insulin under the skin. It is a complete tubing system to connect an insulin pump to the pump user: it includes a subcutaneous cannula, adhesive mount, quick-disconnect, and a pump cartridge connector.

Insulin: a hormone that helps the body use glucose for energy. The beta cells of the pancreas make insulin. When the body cannot make enough insulin, it is taken by injection or through use of an insulin pump.

Insulin pump: A small, computerized device — about the size of a small cell phone — that is worn on a belt or put in a pocket. Insulin pumps have a small flexible tube with a fine needle on the end. The needle is inserted under the skin of the abdomen and taped in place. A carefully measured, steady flow of insulin is released into the body.

Insulin receptors: Areas on the outer part of a cell that allow insulin in the blood to join or bind with the cell. When the cell and insulin bind together, the cell can take glucose from the blood and use it for energy.

Insulin resistance: the body's inability to respond to and use the insulin it produces. Insulin resistance may be linked to obesity, hypertension, and high levels of fat in the blood.

IVF (in virto fertilization): process by which an egg is fertilized by sperm outside the body: in vitro. IVF is a major treatment for infertility when other methods of assisted reproductive technology have failed.

LADA (latent autoimmune diabetes in adults) diabetes: a condition in which Type 1 diabetes develops in adults.

Lantis (insulin glargine): a long-acting basal insulin analogue, marketed by Sanofi-Aventis, given once daily to help control the blood sugar level of those with diabetes.

MRI (magnetic resonance imaging): medical imaging technique used in radiology to visualize internal structures of the body in detail.

Mmol/L: millimoles per liter, a unit of measure that shows the concentration of a substance in a specific amount of fluid. In most of the world, except for the United States, blood glucose test results are reported as mmol/L. In the United States, milligrams per deciliter (mg/dL) is used.

Mg/dL: milligrams per deciliter, a unit of measure that shows the concentration of a substance in a specific amount of fluid. In the United States, blood glucose test results are reported as mg/dL. Medical journals and other countries use millimoles per liter (mmol/L).

Novolog: fast acting insulin analogue marketed by Novo Nordisk.

Pancreas: An organ behind the lower part of the stomach that is about the size of a hand. It makes insulin so the body can use sugar for energy.

Protein: One of three main classes of food. Proteins are made of amino acids, which are called the "building blocks of the cells." Cells need protein to grow and to mend themselves. Protein is found in many foods, like meat, fish, poultry, eggs, legumes, and dairy products.

TSA: Transportation Security Administration develops and enforces guiding principles to maintain the security of the traveling public and continuously set the standard for excellence in transportation security. http://www.tsa.gov/

Type 1 diabetes: a condition characterized by high blood glucose levels caused by a total lack of insulin. Type 1 diabetes occurs when the body's immune system attacks the insulin-producing beta cells in the pancreas and destroys them. The pancreas then produces little or no insulin. Type 1 diabetes develops most often in young people but can appear in adults.

Type 2 diabetes: a condition characterized by high blood glucose levels caused by either a lack of insulin or the body's inability to use insulin efficiently. Type 2 diabetes develops most often in middle-aged and older adults but can appear in young people.

9.3 ~ Sample Medical Information Lists

My Sample Medical Information Sheet

PATIENT: Joanne Milo
                 816 My Street
                 My City, CA 92000

DOB: 01/06/1960

TEL: 949-816-0000

EMAIL   myname@gmail.com

TEL: 949-422-0001 – mobile

FAX: 949-816-0001

DATE: 16 April 2012

ALLERGIES: Penicillin (rash), Sulfa (hives),
                 Doxycycline (headache)

MEDICATIONS: Insulin: Cozmo Insulin Pump, Novolog, 35 – 40 U/day
                  [for Type 1 diabetes]
                  Calcitriol: 0.5 mcg/ once daily / 6 days/wk [for hypoparathyroidism]
                  Calcium Citrate: 500 mg 3x/day **[CRITICAL SUPPLEMENT]**
                  Vit D: 5,000u/day [for hypoparathyroidism
                  Forteo (PTH): Injection 20 mcg every third day [for osteoporosis]
                  Levothyroid: 112 mcg/daily [for hypothyroidism]
                  Zetia: 10 mg/ 4x/week [to lower LDL]
                  Magnesium Citrate: 750 mg/day **[CRITICAL SUPPLEMENT]**
                  Alpha Lipoic Acid: 600 mg dailu [antioxidant supplement]
                  Multi Vitamin
                  Xyzal: as needed for allergies

My Sample Schedule of Medications

PATIENT: Joanne Milo

816 My Street

My City, CA 92000

TEL: 949-816-0000

FAX: 949-816-0001

DOB: 01/06/1960

Essential medications highlighted in bold

Before Breakfast

Synthroid: 125 mcg/daily

With Breakfast

Calcitriol: 0.5 mcg/ once daily / 6 days/wk

Calcium Citrate: 2 capsules – 250 mg

Vit D: 5,000u/day

Magnesium Citrate: 2 capsules, BioCitrateMag

Alpha Lipoic Acid: 600 mg daily

Before Lunch

Calcium Citrate: 2 capsules – 250mg

Magnesium Citrate: 2 capsules – BioCitrateMag

With Lunch

Before Dinner

Calcium Citrate: 2 capsules – 250mg

Magnesium Citrate: 2 capsules – BioCitrateMag

With Dinner

Zetia: 10 mg/ 4x/week

Forteo (PTH): Injection 20 mcg every other day

My Sample Emergency Contact Sheet

PATIENT: Joanne Milo
            816 My Street
            My City, CA 92000
DOB: 01/06/1960
TEL: 949-816-0000
EMAIL   myname@gmail.com
TEL: 949-422-0001 – mobile
FAX: 949-816-0001

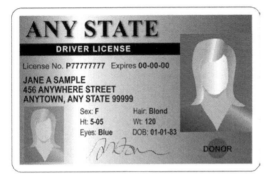

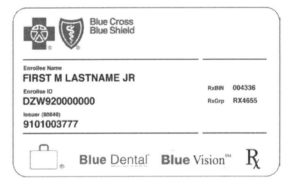

PHYSICIANS

Endocrinologist
Dr. Joseph Ba***
12345 Crown Valley Pkwy
Mission Viejo, CA
949-364-0000
949-364-0000 (fax)

Internist
Dr. David Br***
12345 Hospital Road
Newport Beach, CA
949-574-0000
949-650-0000 (fax)

Ophthalmologist
Dr. Allan Kr***
210 Stein Plaza
Westwood, CA
310 825 0000

EMERGENCY CONTACTS

Richard M**** (spouse)
816 My Street
My City, CA 92000
949-717-0000
949-533-0000 (cell)

Christy J*****
949-375-0000

Donna H*****
949-722-0000 (home)

Dr. Paul & Melissa S*******
949-859-0000 (home)
949-452-0000 (office)
949-280-0000 (cell)

Alexis S******, daughter
949-922-0000 (cell)

Robin & Stan N***
949-725-0000

Pharmacy
RiteAid Bayside Drive
Newport Beach, CA
949-760-1234

Remember, you can be prepared by keeping your *The Savvy Diabetic: On The Go* workbook up-to-date and ready to go, available on www.TheSavvyDiabetic.com.

Blank Form: My Medicine List

From ASHP Foundation, American Society of Health-System Pharmacists

www.ashpfoundation.org

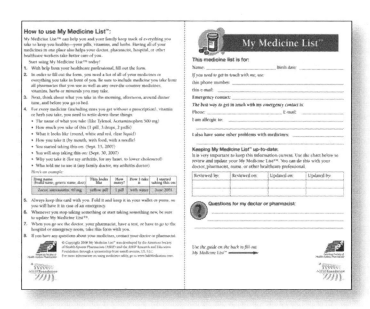

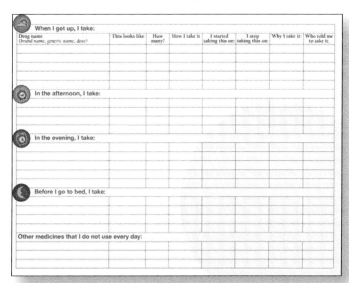

Blank Form and Wallet Card: MedicAlert Foundation

PERSONAL INFORMATION

FIRST NAME   MIDDLE NAME

LAST NAME

MAILING ADDRESS   UNIT/APT #

CITY   STATE   ZIP

PHONE ☐ Home ☐ Cell ☐ Work   ☐ Home ☐ Cell ☐ Work

EMAIL ADDRESS (STRONGLY RECOMMENDED)

☐ Male ☐ Female

DATE OF BIRTH   GENDER

EMERGENCY CONTACTS*

PRIMARY EMERGENCY CONTACT   RELATIONSHIP

EMERGENCY CONTACT'S PHONE   SECOND PHONE

PRIMARY PHYSICIAN   PHYSICIAN PHONE

MEDICAL CONDITIONS/ALLERGIES/MEDICATIONS*

NO KNOWN ☐ MEDICAL CONDITIONS ☐ ALLERGIES ☐ MEDICATIONS

PLEASE GO ONLINE TO COMPLETE YOUR FULL MEDICAL RECORD.
* Please attach additional listings if needed

SELECT YOUR MEMBERSHIP

☐ Kid Smart ($40/yr)   _____
☐ Advantage ($50/yr)   _____
☐ MedicAlert + Safe Return ($55/yr) _____

Essential ($30/3yrs) - Available online only
Advance Directive Management Service ($30/3yrs) - Available online only
Caregiver Membership - Learn more at www.medicalert.org/caregiver
Family Membership - Learn more at www.medicalert.org/family

SELECT YOUR MEDICAL ID(S)

see select medical ID details on back of form or view all medical IDs online
at www.medicalert.org/shopids

ID # _____ Price _____

Wrist size (Please measure your wrist & add ½")   _____
Need measuring tips? Go to www.medicalert.org/sizing

Shipping and handling $7.00

TOTAL   _____

PAYMENT

☐ Check ☐ Money Order
☐ MasterCard* ☐ Visa* ☐ Discover* ☐ AMEX*
No other cards accepted. No CODs. Payment must accompany order.

CREDIT CARD NUMBER   EXPIRATION DATE (MM/YY)

CREDIT CARD HOLDER'S NAME

CREDIT CARD HOLDER'S ADDRESS

SIGNATURE FOR CARD AUTHORIZATION

To ensure uninterrupted MedicAlert membership, your credit card will be
automatically charged the membership renewal rate on your renewal date.

☐ Check the box if you don't want us to charge your credit card for renewal.

Important: By accepting membership in MedicAlert Foundation, for yourself as member or caregiver
and/or as caregiver on behalf of the member named above (collectively, "you"), you authorize
MedicAlert to release all medical and other confidential information to emergency and
to other health care personnel you designate. If you choose to terminate membership, you must
notify us in writing and return your jewelry. MedicAlert relies upon the accuracy of the information
that you provide. You, therefore, agree to defend, indemnify, and hold MedicAlert (including its
employees, officers, directors, agents, and organizations with which it maintains a marketing alliance
for the provision of services hereunder) harmless from any claim or lawsuit brought by another or
others for injury, death, loss or damages arising in whole or in part out of your provision of incomplete
or inaccurate information to MedicAlert. Furthermore, as caregiver for the member named above,
you hereby represent and warrant to MedicAlert that you have full power and authority, as the duly
authorized representative of such member, to enroll and act on his or her behalf.

SIGNATURE OF MEMBER   DATE
(A parent or guardian signature is required for members under the age of 18.)

Prices are subject to change without notice.

◈ MedicAlert
F O U N D A T I O N

Mrs. Karen K Jones

Member Number: 1234567890

Valid Until: October 12, 2015

24/7 Emergency Medical Information Service

1.800.607.2565   **1.800.432.5378**
EMERGENCIES ONLY   MEMBER SERVICES

MedicAlert Foundation is a 501(c)(3) nonprofit organization. ©2012 All rights reserved.
MedicAlert® is a U.S. registered trademark and service mark.

E M E R G E N C Y   I N F O

9.4 ~ Sample Hospital Diet Plans and Menus

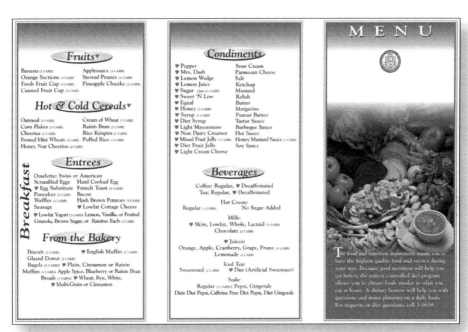

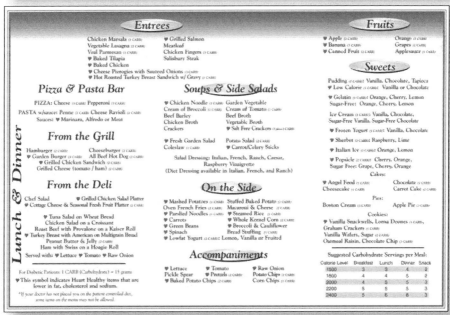

9.5 ~ TSA Information for Travelers, 2013

If a passenger uses an insulin pump, he or she can be screened without disconnecting from the pump. However, it is important for the passenger to inform the Transportation Security Officer (TSO) conducting the screening about the pump before the screening process begins.

TSA has created notification cards that travelers may use to inform TSOs about any disability, medical condition, or medical device that could affect security screening. Although these cards do not exempt anyone from security screening, their use may improve communication and help travelers discreetly notify TSOs of their conditions. This card can be found at:

http://www.tsa.gov sites default files publications disability_notification_cards.pdf.

Passengers can be screened using Advanced Imaging Technology (AIT) only if they can stand still with their arms above their heads for 5-7 seconds without the support of a person or device. Similarly, passengers can be screened using walk-through metal detectors only if they can walk through on their own. An eligible passenger can request to be screened by AIT if it is available or can request to be screened using a thorough pat-down; however, passengers cannot request to be screened by the walk-through metal detector in lieu of AIT or a pat-down.

If a passenger cannot or chooses not to be screened by AIT or a walk-through metal detector, the passenger will be screened using a thorough pat-down procedure instead. A pat-down procedure also is used to resolve any alarms of a metal detector or anomalies identified by AIT. If a pat-down is required in order to complete screening:

The pat-down should be conducted by a TSO of the same gender. Sometimes, passengers must wait for a TSO of the same gender to become available.

The passenger can request a private screening at any time and a private screening should be offered when the TSO must pat-down sensitive areas.

During a private screening, another TSA employee will also be present and the passenger may be accompanied by a companion of his or her choosing.

A passenger may ask for a chair if he or she needs to sit down.

The passenger should inform TSOs of any difficulty raising his or her arms, remaining in the position required for a pat-down, or any areas of the body that are painful when touched.

A passenger should not be asked to remove or lift any article of clothing to reveal a sensitive body area.

In addition to the pat-down, TSA may use technology to test for traces of explosive material. If explosive material is detected, the passenger will have to undergo additional screening. For more information about the technology used to test for traces of explosive material, please visit

Regardless of whether the passenger is screened using AIT or the walk-through metal detector, the passenger's insulin pump is subject to additional screening. Under most circumstances, this will include the passenger conducting a self-pat-down of the insulin pump followed by an explosive trace detection sampling of the passenger's hands.

A companion, assistant, or family member may accompany a passenger to assist him or her during any private or public screening. After providing this assistance, the companion, assistant, or family member will need to be rescreened. The passenger should inform the TSO of his or her need for assistance before the screening process begins.

If a passenger has concerns about his or her screening, he or she should ask to speak with a supervisor while at the checkpoint. Passengers also can report concerns by contacting TSA's Disability and Multicultural Division at TSA.ODPO@tsa.dhs.gov or

> Transportation Security Administration
> Disability and Multicultural Division
> 601 South 12th Street
> Arlington, VA 20598

TSA encourages passengers with disabilities or medical conditions to arrive at the airport early and to visit www.tsa.gov for more information before they fly.

Diabetes-related supplies, medication, equipment (insulin inhalers, glucagon emergency kits, lancets, blood glucose meters and strips, alcohol swabs, meter-testing solutions, urine ketone test strips, insulin pumps, and pump supplies) and used syringes (when transported in a Sharps disposal container or other similar hard-surface container) are allowed through the security checkpoint once they have been properly screened by x-ray or a hand inspection.

Passengers should declare these items and separate them from other belongings for screening.

TSA limits the amount of liquids, gels, or aerosols that passengers can bring through the security screening checkpoint. The 3-1-1 rule states that all liquids, gels, and aerosols must be in 3.4 ounce (100ml) or less (by volume) containers; the containers should be in a 1 quart-sized, clear, plastic, zip-top bag; and 1 bag per passenger can be placed in a screening bin. Medically necessary items are not subject to the 3-1-1 limitation and are allowed through the checkpoint in any amount once they have been screened.

Passengers are encouraged to bring through the checkpoint only the amount of medically necessary liquids or gels they will reasonably need for the duration of their itinerary, allowing for delays, and to pack the rest in checked baggage. Passengers should inform a TSO if a liquid or gel is medically necessary and separate it from other belongings before screening begins.

Liquids, gels, and aerosols are screened by x-ray, and medically necessary items in excess of 3.4 ounces will receive additional screening, which could include screening with bottled liquid screening technologies. Depending on the technology available at the checkpoint, a passenger could be asked to open the liquid or gel for screening. TSA will not touch the liquid or gel during this process. If the passenger does not want a liquid, gel, or aerosol x-rayed or opened, he or she should inform the TSO before screening begins. Additional screening of the passenger and his or her property may be required, which may include a pat-down.

9.6 ~ Foreign Language Translations

"Life is a foreign language: all men mispronounce it."
~ *Christopher Morley, American journalist, novelist, poet*

Here are some examples of the following statement in foreign languages. For more languages, go to www.google.com, and choose Translate, under More. Type in the phrase and choose the language for the countries you will be visiting.

English:

"I have diabetes. I wear an insulin pump. I carry syringes to take insulin, my medication. I wear a device to monitor my blood glucose."

Afrikaans:

Ek het diabetes. Ek het 'n insulien pomp. Ek dra spuite insulien te neem, my medikasie. Ek dra 'n toestel my bloed glukose te monitor.

Chinese:

我患有糖尿病。我穿一个胰岛素泵。我随身携带注射器，胰岛素，我的药物。我穿了设备监测我的血糖。

French:

J'ai le diabète. Je porte une pompe à insuline. Je porte seringues prendre de l'insuline, mon médicament. Je porte un appareil pour contrôler ma glycémie.

German:

Ich habe Diabetes. Ich trage eine Insulinpumpe. Ich trage Spritzen, Insulin zu nehmen, meine Medikamente. Ich trage ein Gerät an meinen Blutzucker überwachen.

Greek:

Έχω διαβήτη. I wewar μια αντλία ινσουλίνης. Κουβαλάω σύριγγες να πάρετε την ινσουλίνη, τα φάρμακά μου. Φοράω μια συσκευή για την παρακολούθηση της γλυκόζης στο αίμα μου.

Spanish:

Tengo diabetes. Me pongo una bomba de insulina. Llevo jeringas a tomar insulina, la medicación. Me pongo un dispositivo para controlar la glucosa en mi sangre.

Italian:

Ho il diabete. Indosso una pompa di insulina. Io porto siringhe di prendere l'insulina, la mia medicina. Indosso un dispositivo per monitorare la glicemia.

Japanese:

私は糖尿病を持っている。私はインスリンポンプを着用してください。私は注射器が、私の薬をインスリンを取るために運ぶ。私は自分の血糖値を監視する装置を着用してください。

Korean:

나는 당뇨병이. 나는 인슐린 펌프를 착용하십시오. 나는 주사기, 내 약을 인슐린을 취할 수행한다. 내 혈당을 모니터링 할 장치를 착용하십시오.

Polish:

Mam cukrzycę. Noszę pompy insulinowej. I nosić strzykawki przyjmować insulinę, moje lekarstwo. I nosić urządzenie do monitorowania mojej glukozy we krwi.

Russian:

У меня диабет. Я ношу инсулиновой помпы. Я несу шприцы принимать инсулин, мое лекарство. Я ношу устройство для контроля глюкозы в крови моей.

Swahili:

Nina ugonjwa wa kisukari. Mimi kuvaa pampu ya insulini. Mimi kubeba sindano kuchukua insulini, dawa zangu. Mimi kuvaa kifaa kufuatilia damu yangu glucose.

Thai:

ฉันมีโรคเบาหวาน ผมใส่อินซูลินปั๊ม ผมพกเข็มฉีดยาที่จะใช้อินซูลินยาของ
ผมสวมใส่อุปกรณ์ในการตรวจสอบระดับน้ำตาลในเลือดของฉัน

Vietnamese:

Tôi mắc bệnh tiểu đường. Tôi mặc một máy bơm insulin. Tôi mang bơm kim tiêm để tiêm insulin, thuốc của tôi. Tôi mặc một thiết bị để theo dõi lượng đường trong máu của tôi.

9.7 ~ Conversion Charts

Blood Glucose Level Conversion Chart

(mg/dl) / 18 = mmol/l

USA units	Int'l Units	USA units	Int'l Units	USA units	Int'l Units
mg / dl	mmol / l	mg / dl	mmol / l	mg / dl	mmol / l
15	0.8	150	8.3	285	15.8
20	1.1	155	8.6	290	16.1
25	1.4	160	8.9	295	16.4
30	1.7	165	9.2		
35	1.9	170	9.4	300	16.7
40	2.2	175	9.7	325	18.1
45	2.5	180	10.0	350	19.4
50	2.8	185	10.3	375	20.8
55	3.1	190	10.6	400	22.2
60	3.3	195	10.8	425	23.6
65	3.6	200	11.1	450	25.0
70	3.9	205	11.4	475	26.4
75	4.2	210	11.7	500	27.8
80	4.4	215	11.9	525	29.2
85	4.7	220	12.2	550	30.6
90	5.0	225	12.5	575	31.9
95	5.3	230	12.8	600	33.3
100	5.6	235	13.1	625	34.7
105	5.8	240	13.3	650	36.1
110	6.1	245	13.6	675	37.5
115	6.4	250	13.9	700	38.9
120	6.7	255	14.2	725	40.3
125	6.9	260	14.4	750	41.7
130	7.2	265	14.7	775	43.1
135	7.5	270	15.0	800	44.4
140	7.8	275	15.3	825	45.8
145	8.1	280	15.6	850	47.2

The Savvy Diabetic: A Survival Guide

Celsius to Fahrenheit Conversion Chart

C = (F -32)*5/9   or   F = (C*9/5) +32

Storage Temp		Body Temp		Body Temp		Storage Temp	
°C	°F	°C	°F	°C	°F	°C	°F
-30	-22	36.0	96.8	38.0	100.4	40	104
-25	-13	36.1	97.0	38.1	100.6	41	106
-20	-4	36.2	97.2	38.2	100.8	42	108
-15	5	36.3	97.3	38.3	100.9	43	109
-10	14	36.4	97.5	38.4	101.1	44	111
-5	23	36.5	97.7	38.5	101.3	45	113
0	32	36.6	97.9	38.6	101.5	50	122
5	41	36.7	98.1	38.7	101.7	55	131
10	50	36.8	98.2	38.8	101.8	60	140
15	59	36.9	98.4	38.9	102.0	65	149
20	68	37.0	98.6	39.0	102.2	70	158
25	77	37.1	98.8	39.1	102.4	75	167
30	86	37.2	99.0	39.2	102.6	80	176
31	88	37.3	99.1	39.3	102.7	85	185
32	90	37.4	99.3	39.4	102.9	90	194
33	91	37.5	99.5	39.5	103.1	95	203
34	93	37.6	99.7	39.6	103.3	100	212
35	95	37.7	99.9	39.7	103.5	105	221
		37.8	100.0	39.8	103.6		
		37.9	100.2	39.9	103.8		
		38.0	100.4	40.0	104.0		

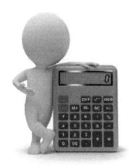

214

Made in the USA
San Bernardino, CA
05 May 2018